NATURAL REM...

FOR ALL KINDS OF

DISEASES: CANCER,

HEART, DIABETES AND

MORE.

Inspired by

Barbara O'Neill's Teachings.

Niella Brown

Disclaimer:

The information provided in this book is for informational purposes only. Please consult with your health care provider for medical advice. The author specifically disclaims any liability that is incurred from the use or application of the contents of this book

Inspired By Barbara O'Neill's Teachings

Get Exclusive Access To all Barbara O'Neill's Videos, Lectures and Teachings.

Scan the Code Below to get Started.

INTRODUCTION

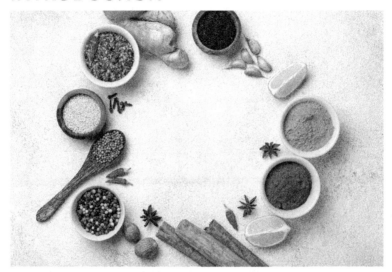

Welcome to a journey of empowerment and enlightenment about health and wellness. "Natural Remedies for All Kinds of Diseases" is not just a book; it's a beacon of hope for those who seek to harness the power of nature in healing and maintaining optimal health. This guide is rooted in the understanding that the body possesses an innate ability to heal itself, given the right conditions and support.

Based on Barbara O'Neill's Teaching

Barbara O'Neill, a renowned naturopath and nutritionist, has long been a proponent of natural remedies for treating a wide range of diseases. Her philosophy centers on the belief that the body, given the right conditions, has an innate ability to heal itself. O'Neill emphasizes the importance of natural healing methods, advocating for a holistic approach to health that combines diet, exercise, and lifestyle changes. This approach reflects a deep respect for the body's natural processes and a commitment to nurturing health from within.

O'Neill's teachings advocate for using food as medicine. She believes that a diet rich in whole, plant-based foods can prevent and even reverse many chronic diseases. Her approach also includes the use of herbs, water therapy, and detoxification methods, all aimed at restoring the body's balance and enhancing its natural healing capabilities.

In her work, O'Neill often emphasizes the importance of understanding the root causes of diseases rather than just treating symptoms. This holistic perspective encourages a deeper awareness of how lifestyle choices impact health and promotes a proactive approach to disease prevention.

Her influence has inspired many to turn to natural remedies as a viable alternative to conventional medicine, highlighting the potential of nature's own resources in maintaining health and wellness. O'Neill's teachings continue to resonate with those seeking a more natural and holistic approach to health care.

Barbara O'Neill's teachings on natural remedies for various diseases:

- **Holistic Health Approach**: Emphasizes treating the whole person, including body, mind, and spirit, rather than just the symptoms of a disease.
- **Food as Medicine**: Advocates a diet rich in whole, plant-based foods to prevent and treat illnesses.
- **Importance of Nutrition**: Stresses the role of vitamins, minerals, and other nutrients in maintaining health and fighting disease.
- **Detoxification**: Encourages natural detox methods such as fasting, herbal remedies, and water therapy to cleanse the body.
- **Herbal Remedies**: Utilizes the healing properties of herbs for various health conditions.
- **Lifestyle Changes**: Recommends lifestyle modifications like adequate sleep, stress

management, and regular physical activity for overall well-being.

- **Water Therapy**: Promotes the use of hydrotherapy as a natural healing method.
- **Gut Health**: Highlights the significance of a healthy gut and digestive system in overall health.
- **Natural Immune Boosters**: Focuses on natural ways to strengthen the immune system.
- **Avoidance of Toxins**: Advises on reducing exposure to environmental and dietary toxins.
- **Self-Care Practices**: Encourages practices like meditation and mindfulness for mental and emotional health.
- **Education and Empowerment**: Aims to educate individuals about their health and empower them to take control of their wellbeing through natural methods.

Understanding Natural Remedies

Natural remedies have stood the test of time, and their relevance in modern times has only flourished amidst our growing desire to take a more active role in our health care. These remedies encompass a broad range of practices and substances used to promote health, from herbs and foods to holistic practices that align body, mind, and spirit.

This book demystifies these practices, providing you with a clear understanding of how natural ingredients and techniques can prevent, alleviate, or even cure diseases. Self-healing is an ancient philosophy that encourages personal responsibility for one's health. It's a concept that recognizes the individual as the primary caretaker of their well-being. This philosophy is grounded in the belief that by making informed decisions about diet, lifestyle, and stress management, one can influence their health outcomes significantly. Through this book, you'll explore how to activate your body's self-healing mechanisms, fostering a balance that promotes long-term health.

How to Use This Book

This book is designed to be your companion and guide, whether you're navigating through a specific health challenge or simply aiming to live a healthier life. Each chapter addresses a different health condition, providing insight into the role natural remedies play in treatment and prevention. The chapters are structured to lead you from understanding the basics to delving into the specifics of each remedy, including how-to steps, dosages, and safety considerations. Additionally, real-life stories and case studies punctuate the text, bringing to life the transformative power of natural healing.

As you turn each page, keep an open mind and remember that the path to health is as individual as you are. Use this book as a starting point for conversations with healthcare professionals and as a resource to develop your personalized health plan. Your body is a remarkable system capable of remarkable things, and with the right knowledge and tools, you can steer it towards a healthier tomorrow.

Embrace this book with the curiosity of a novice and the focus of a scientist. Let's embark on this path together, with nature as our guide and self-healing as our goal.

CHAPTER 1: FOUNDATIONS OF HEALTH

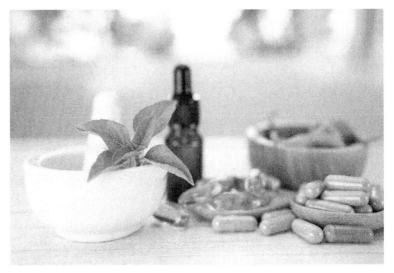

A t the heart of every natural remedy is the principle that the body is designed to heal itself. This is where we begin our journey into the Foundations of Health. To understand how to treat illnesses, we must first understand the essential elements that contribute to overall wellness. These foundations are like the legs of a table—remove one, and the whole structure wobbles. They include nutrition, hydration, sleep, and exercise. By maintaining these core aspects, we can create a robust platform for health that supports the body's intrinsic healing processes.

1. Nutrition: The Building Blocks of Life

Good nutrition is fundamental to good health. The foods we eat provide the energy and nutrients needed to fuel body processes, repair tissue, and regulate vital functions. Whole, unprocessed foods are the keystones of a healthful diet—they are rich in antioxidants, vitamins, and minerals that protect against disease. Understanding the role of macronutrients (carbohydrates, proteins, and fats) and micronutrients (vitamins and minerals) is critical for crafting a diet that supports health rather than undermines it.

2. Hydration: The Essence of Vitality

Our bodies are mostly water, and every system depends on it to function. Water flushes toxins from the body, carries nutrients to cells, provides a moist environment for ear, nose, and throat tissues, and eliminates waste. Without adequate water, nothing in the body operates efficiently, and the risk of health issues—from kidney stones to constipation—increases.

3. Sleep: The Natural Healer

Sleep is not merely a passive state of rest but a dynamic process of restoration and healing. During sleep, the body repairs its muscles and tissues, consolidates memories, and releases hormones that regulate growth and appetite. Chronic sleep deprivation can lead to a host of health problems, including obesity, heart disease, and diabetes. Cultivating good sleep hygiene is, therefore, a critical aspect of maintaining health.

4. Exercise: The Currency of Health

Exercise is the currency with which we buy health. It strengthens the heart, improves circulation, tones muscles, and enhances flexibility. Regular physical activity is linked with a lower risk of chronic diseases such as heart disease, stroke, and type 2 diabetes. It's also vital for mental health, releasing endorphins that reduce stress and improve mood.

By delving into each of these foundations, we can understand how they interact with and support each other. For instance, good nutrition can improve sleep quality, while adequate hydration can enhance the effectiveness of exercise. Conversely, poor management of one can negatively impact the others, creating a domino effect that leads to ill health.

With this overview, we're setting the stage for a deep dive into each component, exploring the science behind why they're vital and how we can optimize them in our lives to prevent, treat, and manage various diseases. The goal is not just to live longer but to live better, with vitality and vigor that comes from a well-nourished, well-rested, and well-exercised body.

Nutrition: The Building Blocks of Life

Nutrition isn't just about eating; it's about feeding every cell in your body the right way. It's about discovering the alchemy of ingredients that can boost our immunity, energize our days, and strengthen our bones. The food we consume can be our most potent medicine or our slowest poison. In this chapter, we will explore the transformative power of nutrition, understanding how the quality of the fuel we provide our bodies influences our overall health and wellness.

The Essence of Nutrition

Nutrition is a science that examines the relationship between diet and health. Essential nutrients include vitamins, minerals, fats, proteins, and carbohydrates — each playing a unique role in maintaining optimal bodily function. Proteins are the body's building materials, used to create and repair tissues, while carbohydrates are the primary energy source for all body functions. Fats are crucial for long-term energy storage, and absorption of certain vitamins, and are integral to cell membrane structure. Vitamins and minerals, although required in smaller amounts, are vital for supporting body processes like blood clotting, energy production, and the immune system.

Macronutrients are nutrients that our bodies need in large amounts. These include carbohydrates, proteins, and fats, each serving a unique purpose. Carbohydrates are the body's main energy source, and getting the right balance of complex carbs (like those found in whole grains and vegetables) is crucial for sustained energy. Proteins are the bodybuilding blocks, crucial for growth and repair. They are not just in meat and beans but are also richly present in nuts and some grains. Fats, often misunderstood, are essential for brain health, energy, and hormone production. The focus is on healthy fats from sources like avocados, nuts, and fish, which can protect the heart and support overall health.

While macronutrients get much of the spotlight, micronutrients—vitamins, minerals, and trace elements—play equally pivotal roles. They're crucial in small quantities for preventing disease, maintaining energy levels, and keeping skin and eyes healthy. We'll touch on the 'silent heroes' like vitamin D for bone health, antioxidants for cellular repair, and iron for blood oxygenation.

Another nutrient often overlooked is water. Often forgotten in nutrition discussions, water is perhaps the most critical nutrient of all. It regulates our body temperature, aids in digestion, and helps flush out toxins. It's the solvent that carries nutrients to cells, and it's vital for kidney function and maintaining electrolyte balance.

The right nutrition goes hand in hand with a balanced lifestyle. It's not just what we eat but how we eat. Stress, sleep, and physical activity levels intertwine with our dietary choices to shape our health. For example, the interplay between diet and sleep is significant, as poor nutrition can lead to sleep disturbances, which in turn can affect dietary choices the next day.

As we go on, it is important to base our diet on a variety of whole foods, rich in the nutrients we've discussed. A well-rounded diet filled with fruits, vegetables, whole grains, lean proteins, and healthy fats is foundational to a lifestyle that promotes vitality and disease prevention. In the next sections, we'll explore how to apply these principles to create a personalized nutrition plan that supports your health and well-being goals.

Hydration: The Essence of Vitality

Hydration, quite simply, is the act of keeping your body adequately supplied with water. Water is crucial because every cell in your body needs it to function properly. It's not just about quenching thirst; hydration influences virtually every physiological process in your body, including circulation, digestion, and temperature regulation.

Let's dive deeper into why hydration is so vital. Your body is about 60% water, and this water is continuously used and must be replenished. You lose water through everyday actions like sweating, breathing, and eliminating waste. Not replacing this water can lead to dehydration, which, even in mild cases, can cause headaches, lethargy, and dry skin. In severe cases, dehydration can lead to more serious complications such as kidney stones or urinary tract infections.

The benefits of staying hydrated are vast. Adequate water intake helps to keep your joints lubricated, preventing the discomfort that comes with wear and tear. It also aids in maintaining a healthy balance of bodily fluids, which can help manage blood pressure and regulate heart rate. Hydration supports the transportation of nutrients and oxygen to cells, keeping your body energized and functioning at its peak.

But how much water should one drink? The "eight glasses a day" rule is a good starting point, but individual needs can vary based on factors such as weight, climate, and activity level. An easy check for hydration is the color of your urine—it should be light yellow. Dark urine often indicates that you need more fluids.

It's also worth noting that hydration isn't just about water intake; it's about how your body uses water. This can be affected by your diet and lifestyle. For example, high intakes of caffeinated or alcoholic beverages can dehydrate you, as can a diet high in salty or sugary foods. On the other hand, eating water-rich foods like cucumbers, oranges, and strawberries can contribute to your hydration levels.

Maintaining hydration is essential for health and vitality. It's not just about drinking water; it's about making sure your body can use that water effectively. So listen to your body, pay attention to the signs it gives you, and keep water close at hand throughout your day. It's a simple step with a profound impact on your well-being.

The Role of Water in the Body

Water is the body's most essential nutrient, a versatile key that unlocks a multitude of biological locks. It's the medium in which all cellular activities occur, from the transportation of nutrients to the elimination of waste. Each cell in our body is a microcosm of life, buoyed and sustained by water's nurturing flow. Below are the roles of water in the body;

- **Transportation:** Highways of blood and lymph fluid are water's domain, carrying life-giving oxygen and nutrients to distant cells and whisking away the refuse of metabolic labor.

- **Chemical Reactions:** Water is the stage for biochemical reactions, the reactant that participates actively in metabolic processes, and the solvent that dissolves and distributes vital compounds.

- **Temperature Regulation:** Like Earth's climate controlled by its oceans, our body's temperature is regulated by water's capacity to absorb and redistribute heat.

- **Lubrication:** Joints swivel and glide in their sockets, cushioned by water-based fluids, while organs are enrobed in moist membranes that protect and provide structure.

Hydration and Health

Staying well-hydrated is likened to keeping a river flowing smoothly in its banks—too little, and the riverbed cracks, too much, and the waters overstep their bounds. Proper hydration supports health by:

- **Enhancing Physical Performance:** Muscles bathed in sufficient water contract with vigor, and endurance soars. Dehydration can lead to fatigue, reduced motivation, and increased susceptibility to heat stress.

- **Boosting Cognitive Function:** A hydrated brain is a swift and agile mind. Cognitive functions such as concentration, alertness, and memory can all suffer when dehydration creeps in.

- **Supporting Digestion and Weight Management:** Water helps dissolve fibers and allows for the smooth passage of food through the digestive tract. It also plays a role in satiety and can aid in weight management efforts.

- **Detoxification:** The kidneys, nature's filtration system, rely on water to flush out soluble waste and toxins through urine.

- **Skin Health:** Like a grape's smooth surface compared to a raisin's wrinkles, our skin reflects our hydration levels, with adequate water contributing to a healthy, glowing complexion.

Strategies for Adequate Hydration

Hydration is not a one-size-fits-all recipe. The amount of water needed can vary based on age, weight, climate, activity level, and individual health conditions. Here are some strategies to stay hydrated:

- **Listen to Your Body:** Thirst is the body's SOS for water. Drinking to quench thirst is a basic yet effective strategy.

- **Eat Water-Rich Foods:** Fruits and vegetables like cucumbers, oranges, and watermelons are juicy allies in the quest for hydration.

- **Monitor the Signs:** Clear urine and regular bathroom breaks are good indicators of proper hydration.

- **Make a Routine:** Start with a glass of water in the morning and keep a bottle handy throughout the day.

- **Spice Up Your Water:** A slice of lemon, a sprig of mint, or a splash of juice can make hydration more enjoyable.

Hydration is the cornerstone of a thriving body and mind. It's a simple yet profound act of nourishment that's easily incorporated into daily life, bringing a wellspring of health benefits. As we understand and respect the role of water in our well-being, we unlock the potential to elevate our health to its highest tide. Drink up—the essence of vitality awaits in each sip.

Sleep: The Natural Healer

Sleep, often overlooked in the hustle of modern life, is an indispensable part of the human health puzzle. It's not just about recharging energy;

it's a complex restorative process that supports cognitive function, emotional balance, and overall physical health. Understanding sleep's multifaceted role can empower us to treat it with the same respect we give to diet and exercise.

The Essential Roles of Sleep

Sleep serves numerous vital functions:

- **Cellular Repair and Growth:** During deep sleep, the growth hormone is released, aiding in cell repair and growth. This process is crucial for recovering from the day's wear and tear.

- **Cognitive Maintenance:** Sleep consolidates memories and facilitates learning. Without adequate sleep, our ability to focus, make decisions, and learn new information plummets.

- **Metabolic Health:** Sleep regulates hormones that control appetite and insulin sensitivity, playing a key role in weight management and the risk of diabetes.

- **Emotional Regulation:** Adequate sleep helps to balance mood and emotions, reducing the risk of conditions like depression and anxiety.

- **Immune System Function:** Sleep boosts the immune system, which helps to fend off infections and even has implications in cancer prevention.

The Healing Power of Sleep

In the context of disease, sleep's restorative power is even more pronounced. For those facing illnesses such as cancer, heart disease, or diabetes, sleep can play a role in managing symptoms and improving outcomes.

- **Cancer:** Research suggests that good sleep can support cancer treatments by maintaining a robust immune response and possibly reducing the growth rate of tumors.

- **Heart Disease:** Sleep affects blood pressure and cholesterol levels, two significant risk factors for heart disease. Quality sleep can help to keep these in check.

- **Diabetes:** Proper sleep patterns help to regulate the hormones that affect blood sugar levels, supporting diabetes management.

Creating a Sleep-Positive Environment

To harness the healing power of sleep, one must create the right environment and adopt practices that promote restful sleep:

- **Consistent Schedule:** Going to bed and waking up at the same time every day sets a rhythm for the body's internal clock.

- **Sleep Hygiene:** Keeping the bedroom dark, quiet, and cool can signal to the body that it's time to wind down.

- **Pre-Sleep Routine:** Engaging in relaxing activities before bed, like reading or taking a warm bath, can prepare the mind and body for sleep.

- **Diet and Exercise:** Regular physical activity and a balanced diet can improve sleep quality, but timing is key. Avoiding caffeine before bedtime and heavy meals can make a significant difference.

Sleep Disorders and Remedies

However, achieving restorative sleep isn't always straightforward. Sleep disorders like insomnia, sleep apnea, and restless leg syndrome can disrupt this healing process. Natural remedies, such as valerian root, melatonin supplements, and magnesium, have been researched for their potential to support better sleep.

Integrating Sleep into a Holistic Health Regimen

Sleep's importance should be woven through every chapter of a natural health guide. It interacts with every aspect of well-being discussed, from the food we eat to the stress we manage. By placing sleep at the center of a holistic health strategy, it's possible to enhance the efficacy of other natural remedies and lifestyle changes.

In summary, sleep is not just a timeout from daily life. It is a state of intense biological activity, underpinning our health and healing capacities. By prioritizing and understanding sleep, we unlock its power as a natural healer, making it an ally in our quest for wellness and a vital component of any natural remedy plan

Exercise: The Currency of Health

Exercise is often hailed as one of the most effective ways to maintain and improve health. Its benefits are far-reaching and can impact every aspect of our well-being. When we exercise, we're not just burning calories or building muscle; we're engaging in a transformative process that affects our body at a cellular level.

Exercise as a Health Essential

Let's break it down: think of your body as an economy. Just as any economy has a currency that keeps it running, the currency for your body's health economy is exercise. It keeps the flow going, ensuring that everything from blood to nutrients gets where it needs to go. It's an investment in the proper functioning of your heart, lungs, muscles, brain, and even mood.

Benefits of Exercise

Regular physical activity can reduce the risk of chronic diseases such as heart disease, diabetes, and certain types of cancer. It's known to help control weight, strengthen bones and muscles, and improve mental health and mood. For instance, when you engage in physical activity, your body releases chemicals called endorphins, which are the body's natural mood lifters.

1. **As a Disease Prevention**

Studies show that moderate to vigorous exercise can boost the immune system's defenses. For cardiovascular health, regular exercise helps improve heart function, lowers blood pressure, and improves cholesterol profiles. It increases insulin sensitivity, which is beneficial for diabetes management and helps manage blood sugar levels more effectively.

2. As a Treatment Adjunct

In the context of diseases like diabetes, heart conditions, and even cancer, exercise acts not just as a preventative measure but also as a complementary treatment. It can alleviate symptoms, improve prognoses, and enhance the quality of life. For example, cancer patients often find that exercise improves fatigue, anxiety, and self-esteem.

Finding the Right Exercise for You

Exercise isn't a one-size-fits-all solution. It's important to find an activity that fits your lifestyle, interests, and health status. Whether it's walking, swimming, yoga, or weightlifting, the best exercise is the one you'll perform consistently. Even everyday activities like gardening or taking the stairs count toward your exercise currency.

Many people find it challenging to start or stick with an exercise routine due to time constraints, lack of interest, or physical limitations. It's crucial to address these barriers by finding creative solutions such as short workouts, finding an exercise buddy, or choosing low-impact exercises if joint pain is a concern.

In conclusion, exercise is a cornerstone of a healthy lifestyle. It's a powerful tool that's available to virtually everyone, and it can be tailored to fit individual needs and circumstances. Like any currency, the more you invest in exercise, the richer you become in health. Starting with small steps and gradually increasing activity can yield substantial health dividends over time.

CHAPTER 3: THE HEALING POWER OF FOODS

The concept that food can be a potent tool for healing is not new, but it is increasingly backed by scientific research. A diet rich in certain foods can prevent, alleviate, or even reverse certain medical conditions. This comprehensive exploration will shed light on how food functions as medicine for various health challenges.

Superfoods for Immunity

Our immune system is a complex network of cells and proteins that defend the body against infection. To function optimally, it requires a variety of nutrients that can often be found in so-called superfoods. These foods contain a concentrated amount of vitamins, minerals, and antioxidants that support immune function.

To boost immunity, one must look beyond vitamin supplements and consider whole foods that pack a punch against pathogens. For example:

- **Citrus fruits** like grapefruits, oranges, and lemons are high in vitamin C, a well-known immune system booster.

- **Red bell peppers** outshine even citrus fruits in terms of vitamin C content and are also rich in beta-carotene.

- **Broccoli** is loaded with vitamins A, C, and E, as well as fiber and many other antioxidants.

- **Garlic** has a long history of use for fighting infections and is also believed to slow down artery hardening.

- **Ginger** can help decrease inflammation, which can reduce sore throat and other inflammatory illnesses.

- **Spinach** is not only rich in vitamin C but also packed with numerous antioxidants and beta carotene, which increases the infection-fighting capability of our immune systems.

- **Yogurt** with live and active cultures (like Greek yogurt) can stimulate your immune system to help fight diseases.

Anti-Inflammatory Foods

Chronic inflammation is associated with many health conditions, from heart disease to arthritis to Alzheimer's. To combat this, a diet rich in anti-inflammatory foods is essential. Omega-3 fatty acids, found in fish like salmon and plant sources like flaxseed, are well-known for their anti-inflammatory effects. They work by reducing the production of molecules and substances linked to inflammation. Anti-inflammatory foods can help:

- **Tomatoes** are a good source of lycopene, which reduces inflammation in the lungs and throughout the rest of the body.

- **Olive oil** provides the body with a healthy dose of fat that can reduce inflammation, mimicking the effects of ibuprofen.

- **Leafy greens**, including spinach, kale, and collards, are high in vitamin E, which plays a key role in protecting the body from pro-inflammatory molecules called cytokines.

- **Nuts** like almonds and walnuts are high in vitamins, including Vitamin E, which can protect the body against inflammation.

Foods That Fight Cancer

Certain foods have been identified to contain cancer-fighting properties. These foods contain a variety of antioxidants and phytochemicals that can help prevent the formation of cancer by protecting cells from damage. Cruciferous vegetables like broccoli and Brussels sprouts are rich in glucosinolates, which studies suggest may play a role in reducing the risk of cancer. Certain foods contain powerful compounds that may help prevent cancer:

- **Cruciferous vegetables** such as broccoli, cabbage, and Brussels sprouts may help protect against cancer due to their high glucosinolate content.

- **Berries** are rich in antioxidants, which protect your cells from free-radical damage associated with cancer.

- **Carrots** contain beta-carotene, an antioxidant that has been linked to reduced rates of certain types of cancer, including stomach cancer.

- **Beans** are high in fiber and have been shown in studies to help protect against colorectal cancer.

- **Whole grains** contain fiber, which may also lower your cancer risk.

Heart-Healthy Foods

Maintaining heart health is paramount for longevity and wellbeing. Heart-healthy foods are those that contribute to the maintenance of healthy blood vessels and a regular heartbeat. Foods rich in soluble fiber, like oats, can help lower cholesterol levels by binding to it in the digestive system and removing it from the body. A heart-healthy diet can help reduce the risk of heart disease and stroke:

- **Whole grains** are a good source of soluble and insoluble fiber, which helps to control blood cholesterol levels.

- **Berries** are also rich in heart-healthy antioxidants and phytonutrients.

- **Avocados** are a source of healthy fats, which can help manage cholesterol.

- **Fish** high in omega-3 fatty acids, like salmon and mackerel, are proven to lower triglycerides and blood pressure.

- **Nuts** and seeds contain omega-3s, fiber, and vitamin E, which can help lower your risk of heart disease.

Dietary Strategies for Diabetes Management

Diabetes management through diet involves controlling blood sugar levels to prevent spikes and crashes. Foods with a low glycemic index, such as lentils, certain fruits, and non-starchy vegetables, have a more gradual effect on blood sugar. Fiber-rich foods are particularly important, as fiber slows carbohydrate digestion and sugar absorption, promoting a more gradual rise in blood sugar. A diet for diabetes management focuses on controlling blood glucose levels through a well-balanced intake of nutrients:

- **Fiber-rich foods** slow sugar absorption and help control blood sugar levels. Beans, whole grains, and legumes are excellent sources of fiber.

- **Fruits and vegetables** provide a bounty of vitamins, minerals, fiber, and antioxidants but should be consumed in moderation due to sugar content.

- **Lean meats** and plant-based proteins help manage weight and improve insulin sensitivity.

- **Healthy fats** from nuts, seeds, avocados, and olive oil can help to slow the absorption of glucose into the bloodstream.

Dietary management for diabetes also involves meal timing, consistent carbohydrate intake, and careful monitoring of blood sugar levels.

By integrating these foods into a balanced diet, one can take significant strides toward preventing and managing chronic diseases.

CHAPTER 4: HERBAL MEDICINE

Herbal medicine, often known as phytotherapy, is the use of plants and plant extracts to promote health and treat illnesses. It's one of the oldest forms of healthcare known to mankind and forms a key part of traditional medicine systems worldwide. Today, it's gaining popularity again as people seek natural, holistic approaches to health.

Origins and Evolution

Herbal medicine dates back thousands of years. Ancient civilizations in Egypt, China, and India documented their use of plants for medicinal purposes. Over time, this knowledge expanded, forming a significant part of traditional healing practices across different cultures.

In herbal medicine, every part of the plant - leaves, roots, flowers, and berries - can be used. These parts are either consumed directly, made into teas, or extracted into tinctures, capsules, and powders. The idea is that plants contain natural substances that can promote health and alleviate illness.

Modern Research and Acceptance

Modern science has begun to recognize the value of herbs. Numerous studies have isolated active compounds in plants that have medicinal properties. For example, the heart medication digoxin was originally derived from the foxglove plant. This growing body of research is helping to integrate herbal medicine more into conventional healthcare.

Common Herbs and Uses

Some well-known herbs include:

1. **Ginger:** Often used for its anti-nausea properties.

2. **Turmeric:** Known for its anti-inflammatory and antioxidant effects.

3. **Ginkgo Biloba:** Used to improve cognitive function.

4. **Echinacea:** Popular for boosting the immune system.

Herbs for Specific Conditions

For cancer, herbs like turmeric and green tea have shown promise due to their antioxidant properties. For heart health, hawthorn and garlic are favored for their ability to support cardiovascular function.

For diabetes, cinnamon and fenugreek might help regulate blood sugar levels.

While herbal medicine can be effective, it's important to approach it with care. Not all herbs are safe for everyone, and some can interact with conventional medications. It's crucial to consult with a healthcare provider before starting any herbal regimen, especially for those with existing health conditions or those who are pregnant or breastfeeding.

Herbal medicine offers a rich and diverse approach to health and wellness. As research continues to evolve, we're likely to see more integration of these natural remedies into mainstream healthcare, offering a more holistic approach to treating and preventing diseases. However, safety and informed use remains paramount.

Herbs for Cancer Support

While herbs are not a cure for cancer, they can play a supportive role in cancer care. Some herbs are known to boost the immune system, reduce the side effects of conventional cancer treatments, and improve overall quality of life.

1. **Turmeric (Curcumin)**: Known for its anti-inflammatory properties, curcumin, the

active component in turmeric, has been studied for its potential to reduce the growth of cancer cells.

2. **Ginger**: Often used to alleviate nausea, a common side effect of chemotherapy.

3. **Milk Thistle**: Believed to have liver-protective qualities, which can be beneficial for patients undergoing certain types of chemotherapy.

Heart-Friendly Herbs

Herbs can be part of a heart-healthy lifestyle. Some may help manage blood pressure, reduce cholesterol levels, and support overall cardiovascular health.

1. **Hawthorn**: Traditionally used for heart-related conditions, it's believed to improve circulation and lower blood pressure.

2. **Garlic**: Known for its cholesterol-lowering effects.

3. **Flaxseed**: Rich in omega-3 fatty acids, beneficial for heart health.

Managing Blood Sugar Naturally

Certain herbs have shown potential in helping to regulate blood sugar levels, which is crucial for managing diabetes and prediabetes.

1. **Cinnamon**: Studies suggest that cinnamon can help lower blood sugar levels.

2. **Fenugreek**: Known to improve glycemic control.

3. **Gymnema Sylvestre**: Often used in Ayurvedic medicine, it may help reduce sugar cravings and lower blood sugar levels.

Safety and Efficacy of Herbal Remedies

Navigating Herbal Medicine Safely While herbs are natural, they are not always safe for everyone. It's essential to consider the following:

- **Consult Healthcare Providers**: Always consult with a healthcare professional before starting any herbal regimen, especially if you have existing health conditions or are on medication.

- **Quality and Purity**: Choose high-quality products from reputable sources to ensure purity and potency.

- **Side Effects and Interactions**: Be aware of potential side effects and interactions with other medications.

The efficacy of herbal remedies can vary. While many herbs have been used traditionally for various ailments, scientific research on their effectiveness is ongoing. It's important to approach herbal medicine with an open mind but also a critical eye, relying on evidence-based information.

In summary, herbal medicine offers a rich tapestry of options for supporting health and treating illnesses. Its integration into modern healthcare requires a balanced approach, respecting traditional wisdom while adhering to contemporary scientific standards. With careful consideration and professional guidance, herbs can be a valuable addition to one's health regimen.

CHAPTER 5: DETOXIFICATION AND CLEANSING: A GATEWAY TO ENHANCED HEALTH

Introduction to Detoxification and Cleansing

In today's world, our bodies are constantly exposed to a variety of toxins, from environmental pollutants to additives in our food. These unwanted substances can accumulate in our bodies, potentially leading to health issues over time. This is where detoxification and cleansing come into play, offering a pathway to flush out these toxins and promote overall health and well-being.

Why Detoxify?

Detoxification is not just a health trend; it's a biological response. Our bodies naturally detoxify every day as part of normal body processes. However, the increased exposure to toxins in modern life can overwhelm these natural systems. Detoxification aids in supporting these natural processes, helping to:

- Enhance the body's natural detoxification systems.

- Improve energy levels and mental clarity.

- Strengthen immune function.

- Improve digestion and gut health.

- Support overall wellness and disease prevention.

Methods of Detoxification

Detoxification methods vary widely, but they typically focus on easing the toxic burden on the body. Some popular methods include:

- **Fasting:** Temporarily abstaining from food, which may give the digestive system a rest and help in toxin elimination.

- **Juice Cleanses:** Consuming only fruit and vegetable juices for a short period to provide the body with nutrients while promoting detoxification.

- **Water Therapy:** Drinking increased amounts of water, sometimes infused with herbs or fruits, to flush toxins from the body.

- **Sweating:** Using saunas or engaging in physical exercise to encourage toxin elimination through sweat.

- **Colon Cleansing:** Techniques such as enemas or colonic irrigation to clean the colon and improve digestive health.

The Detoxifying Foods

Certain foods are known for their detoxifying properties. Including these in your diet can support the body's natural detoxification processes:

- **Leafy Greens:** Spinach, kale, and other greens are high in chlorophyll, which helps cleanse the body.

- **Cruciferous Vegetables:** Broccoli, cauliflower, and Brussels sprouts support liver function and detoxification.

- **Fruits:** Berries, apples, and citrus fruits are rich in antioxidants and fiber, aiding in toxin removal.

- **Garlic and Onions:** These contain sulfur compounds that help the liver detoxify.

- **Green Tea:** Rich in antioxidants, it supports detoxification and enhances liver function.

Detoxification Programs and Protocols

There are numerous detox programs and protocols, each with its approach. Some focus on specific diets, while others incorporate lifestyle changes and supplements. Key considerations for a detox program include:

- **Duration:** Most programs range from a few days to several weeks.

- **Dietary Guidelines:** These often emphasize organic, whole foods and eliminate processed foods, sugars, and alcohol.

- **Supplemental Support:** Some programs include supplements like milk thistle or dandelion root to support liver health.

- **Lifestyle Changes:** Stress reduction, improved sleep, and regular exercise are often part of detox protocols.

Safety and Effectiveness

While detoxification can offer health benefits, it's crucial to approach it safely. Extreme detox diets or prolonged fasting can have adverse effects. It's always advisable to consult with a healthcare professional before starting any detox program, especially for individuals with health conditions or those taking medication.

Detoxification and cleansing practices can be a valuable addition to a healthy lifestyle. By understanding and applying these methods appropriately, one can support their body's natural ability to cleanse itself, leading to improved health and vitality. However, it's important to remember that detoxification is just one aspect of a holistic approach to health. Regular exercise, a balanced diet, and adequate sleep are equally important in maintaining overall well-being.

CHAPTER 6: STRESS MANAGEMENT TECHNIQUES

Stress is an inevitable part of life, but how we manage it can significantly impact our health. Chronic stress has been linked to a range of diseases, including heart disease, diabetes, and mental health disorders. Understanding the role of stress in disease and learning effective stress management techniques can greatly enhance our overall well-being.

The Role of Stress in Disease

Stress, especially when chronic, can wreak havoc on our bodies. It triggers a cascade of hormonal changes, including the release of cortisol and adrenaline, which prepare the body for a "fight or flight" response. While this response is beneficial in acute situations, chronic activation can lead to detrimental effects on various body systems. Prolonged stress has been linked to a weakened immune system, increased risk of cardiovascular diseases, exacerbation of existing conditions like asthma, and can contribute to mental health issues like anxiety and depression.

Natural Stress Relief Strategies

Managing stress effectively often involves lifestyle changes and natural techniques:

1. **Physical Activity**: Regular exercise is one of the most effective stress busters. It not only helps in releasing endorphins (natural mood lifters) but also aids in better sleep, which can be disrupted by stress.

2. **Healthy Diet**: A balanced diet, rich in antioxidants and essential nutrients, supports overall health and helps the body cope better with stress. Foods rich in magnesium, omega-3 fatty acids, and vitamin C are known to reduce stress levels.

3. **Adequate Sleep**: Good sleep hygiene is essential for managing stress. Establishing a regular sleep routine, avoiding caffeine and screens before bedtime, and creating a relaxing bedtime environment can improve sleep quality.

4. **Mindfulness and Meditation**: Practices like mindfulness and meditation can help calm the mind, reduce stress hormones, and improve emotional well-being.

5. **Social Support**: Maintaining a supportive network of friends and family can provide emotional support and a sense of belonging, which can help in coping with stress.

Relaxation Techniques: From Breathing to Meditation

1. **Deep Breathing**: Simple yet powerful, deep breathing can help activate the body's relaxation response. Techniques like diaphragmatic breathing, where you focus on filling the abdomen rather than the chest with air, can be particularly effective.

2. **Progressive Muscle Relaxation**: This involves tensing and then relaxing different muscle groups in the body. It helps in reducing physical tension and mental anxiety.

3. **Guided Imagery**: Involves visualizing a peaceful scene or series of experiences in the mind. This can help shift focus away from stress.

4. **Mindfulness Meditation**: This practice involves staying present and fully engaging with the here and now. It can be done anywhere and involves observing thoughts and sensations without judgment.

5. **Yoga and Tai Chi**: These ancient practices combine physical postures, breathing

exercises, and meditation to enhance overall health and reduce stress.

Balancing Hormones Naturally

Chronic stress can disrupt hormonal balance, leading to issues like fatigue, weight gain, and mood disorders. Natural ways to balance hormones include:

- **Regular Exercise**: Helps in regulating hormones like insulin and cortisol.

- **Healthy Fats**: Incorporating healthy fats like avocados, nuts, and seeds can support hormone production.

- **Reducing Sugar and Refined Carbs**: These can cause imbalances in insulin and other hormones.

- **Stress Management Practices**: Activities like meditation and yoga can help in reducing cortisol levels.

- **Adequate Sleep**: Sleep plays a critical role in the regulation of various hormones, including growth hormone and cortisol.

By incorporating these stress management techniques into our daily lives, we can not only reduce the harmful effects of stress but also improve our overall health and quality of life. Remember, managing stress is not about eliminating it completely but about learning how to respond to it in a healthier way.

CHAPTER 7: ALTERNATIVE THERAPIES

When we talk about alternative therapies, we're diving into a world of healing practices that stand outside the realm of conventional Western medicine. These therapies are often rooted in holistic principles, focusing on treating the whole person — body, mind, and spirit — rather than just the symptoms of a disease. They're about balancing the body's natural healing mechanisms, rather than directly combating illness.

Acupuncture and Acupressure

Acupuncture is a gem in the crown of traditional Chinese medicine. It involves the insertion of very thin needles through your skin at strategic points on your body, known as acupuncture points. This process is believed to rebalance the flow of energy (Qi) in your body. Western scientists think it may stimulate nerves, muscles, and connective tissue, boosting your body's natural painkillers and increasing blood flow.

Acupressure, a cousin to acupuncture, doesn't rely on needles. Instead, it involves applying pressure to specific points on the body using fingers, palms, elbows, or special devices. It's based on the same principles as acupuncture, aiming to stimulate the body's natural self-curative abilities. Acupressure is often used for managing pain, reducing stress, and improving overall well-being.

Chiropractic and Physical Therapies

Chiropractic care focuses on disorders of the musculoskeletal system and the nervous system, and the effects of these disorders on general health. Chiropractors use hands-on spinal manipulation and other alternative treatments, under the belief that proper alignment of the body's musculoskeletal structure, particularly the spine, will enable the body to heal itself without surgery or medication. Manipulation is used to restore mobility to joints restricted by tissue injury.

Physical therapies, broadly speaking, encompass various techniques that use movements and manipulative therapies to improve function and manage pain. This includes exercises, stretching, massage, and the use of equipment like ultrasound or hot and cold therapy. The goal is to enhance mobility, reduce pain, and improve overall fitness and health.

Homeopathy and Naturopathy

Homeopathy is based on the principle of "like cures like." It uses tiny amounts of natural substances, like plants and minerals, to stimulate the healing process. A core belief is that a substance that causes symptoms in a healthy person can, in a very small dose, treat those same symptoms of illness.

Naturopathy, or naturopathic medicine, is a form of alternative medicine that employs an array of pseudoscientific practices branded as "natural" and as promoting "self-healing," including homeopathy, herbalism, and acupuncture, as well as diet and lifestyle counseling.

Each of these therapies offers a unique approach to health and healing, often complementing conventional medical treatments. They're part of a growing recognition of the importance of treating the whole person — mind, body, and spirit — in the pursuit of optimal health and wellness. While some are backed by more scientific research than others, they all share a common goal: to promote healing and improve quality of life in a holistic, non-invasive way.

As with any treatment, it's important to consult with healthcare professionals before starting any alternative therapy, especially if you have existing health conditions or are taking other medications.

CHAPTER 8: SPECIAL TOPICS IN NATURAL REMEDIES

Managing Chronic Pain Naturally

Chronic pain, a persistent and often debilitating condition, affects millions worldwide. Unlike acute pain, which is a temporary discomfort signaling a specific injury or illness, chronic pain lingers, often without a clear cause. It can stem from ongoing conditions such as arthritis, or nerve damage, or be a residual effect of past injuries. The quest for relief leads many to explore natural remedies as an alternative or complement to conventional pain management.

1. **Lifestyle Modifications**: Sometimes, small changes in daily habits can significantly impact chronic pain. Regular low-impact exercise, like swimming or yoga, can improve muscle strength and flexibility, reducing pain. Adequate sleep and stress management techniques, such as meditation or deep-breathing exercises, also play a crucial role.

2. **Dietary Approaches**: Certain foods have anti-inflammatory properties, which can help in managing pain. Including omega-3-

rich foods like fish, flaxseeds, and walnuts, and antioxidants found in berries, nuts, and green leafy vegetables can be beneficial. Simultaneously, reducing processed foods and sugars that can exacerbate inflammation is advised.

3. **Herbal Remedies**: Herbs like turmeric, ginger, and willow bark have been used for centuries for pain relief. They contain compounds that may reduce inflammation and offer relief from pain. However, it's essential to consult with a healthcare professional before starting any herbal supplement, especially if you're on other medications.

4. **Physical Therapies**: Techniques such as acupuncture, massage, and chiropractic care can provide significant relief for some individuals. These therapies can help alleviate muscle tension, improve circulation, and stimulate the body's natural pain-relieving mechanisms.

Skin Health: Natural Approaches

Skin, the body's largest organ, acts as a barrier against environmental threats and regulates temperature and hydration. Skin health is influenced by numerous factors, including diet, stress, and exposure to toxins. Natural approaches to skin health often focus on nurturing the skin from both the inside and outside.

1. **Nutrition for Skin Health**: A diet rich in vitamins, minerals, and antioxidants is vital for healthy skin. Foods high in Vitamin C (like oranges and bell peppers), Vitamin E (like almonds and sunflower seeds), and Omega-3 fatty acids (like salmon and avocados) support skin health.

2. **Natural Skin Care Products**: Using products with natural ingredients can be gentler on the skin. Ingredients like aloe vera, coconut oil, and shea butter are known for their soothing and moisturizing properties. Avoiding harsh chemicals and fragrances can also reduce skin irritation and dryness.

3. **Hydration and Sun Protection**: Drinking plenty of water and protecting the skin from the sun are fundamental for maintaining skin health. Using sunscreens with natural ingredients and wearing protective clothing can prevent sun damage, which is a leading cause of skin aging and problems.

Gut Health and Its Impact on Disease

The gut, also known as the gastrointestinal system, plays a critical role in overall health. It's not just about digestion; the gut is home to a vast community of bacteria, collectively known as the gut microbiome. This microbiome impacts everything from immunity to mental health and has been linked to various diseases.

1. **Diet and the Microbiome**: A diet rich in fiber, fermented foods, and diverse plant-based foods supports a healthy microbiome. Foods like yogurt, kefir, sauerkraut, and fiber-rich fruits and vegetables encourage the growth of beneficial bacteria.

2. **Probiotics and Prebiotics**: Probiotics are live beneficial bacteria found in certain foods and supplements. Prebiotics are fibers that feed these good bacteria. Together, they help maintain gut balance, crucial for digestion, nutrient absorption, and immune function.

3. **Gut Health and Disease Prevention**: Research shows that an unhealthy gut can contribute to a wide range of diseases, including diabetes, obesity, rheumatoid arthritis, and even mental health disorders

like depression and anxiety. Maintaining a healthy gut is, therefore, integral to overall health and disease prevention.

In each of these areas, the approach is to look at the body holistically, understanding that natural remedies often work best in conjunction with a healthy lifestyle. It's crucial to remember that while natural remedies can offer significant benefits, they are not a substitute for professional medical advice or treatment. Always consult healthcare professionals, especially in cases of severe or chronic conditions.

CHAPTER 9: NATURAL REMEDIES FOR CANCER

Cancer, a disease characterized by the uncontrolled growth and spread of abnormal cells, is a multifaceted condition that requires a comprehensive approach to treatment and management. While conventional medicine offers surgery, chemotherapy, and radiation therapy, an increasing number of patients and healthcare practitioners are exploring the role of natural remedies in cancer care. These natural approaches aim to strengthen the body's innate healing capacity, improve quality of life, and complement traditional treatments.

Understanding Cancer and its Natural Therapies

Cancer, in its myriad forms, is not just a physical ailment but also a condition that affects patients emotionally and spiritually. Natural therapies focus on treating the whole person, not just the disease. They encompass a range of practices, from dietary changes to herbal medicine, that aim to detoxify the body, boost the immune system, and provide essential nutrients.

Herbs such as turmeric, known for its active compound curcumin, have shown promise in laboratory studies for their anti-cancer properties. Similarly, green tea, rich in antioxidants, may have a protective effect. However, it's crucial to understand that while these natural agents show potential, they should not replace conventional cancer treatments but rather may be used in conjunction to support overall health.

Integrative Approaches to Cancer Treatment

Integrative oncology is a patient-centered field that combines traditional medical treatments with complementary therapies. This approach seeks to optimize health, quality of life, and clinical outcomes across the cancer care continuum. It involves a team approach, including oncologists, dietitians, psychotherapists, and alternative therapy practitioners, working together to provide a tailored treatment plan for each patient.

For instance, acupuncture has been used to alleviate chemotherapy-induced nausea and pain. Similarly, massage therapy and yoga can help reduce stress and improve the quality of life for cancer patients.

Nutritional Support for Cancer Patients

Nutrition plays a pivotal role in cancer care. A diet rich in fruits, vegetables, whole grains, and lean proteins can provide essential nutrients, support immune function, and help the body cope with the side effects of cancer treatments. Foods high in antioxidants, like berries and leafy greens, are particularly beneficial. Omega-3 fatty acids, found in fish and flaxseeds, may also have anti-inflammatory properties that are beneficial for cancer patients.

Cancer patients need to consult with a dietitian specialized in oncology to tailor dietary approaches according to individual needs and treatment plans.

Mind-Body Practices for Cancer

Mind-body practices encompass a variety of techniques aimed at enhancing the mind's capacity to affect bodily function and symptoms. Techniques like meditation, yoga, and Tai Chi can help reduce stress, alleviate treatment side effects, improve mental clarity, and enhance overall well-being.

Meditation, for instance, has been shown to reduce anxiety and improve the quality of sleep in cancer patients. Support groups and counseling can also play a vital role in providing emotional support, which is an integral part of the healing process.

In conclusion, while natural remedies for cancer offer a holistic approach to support and complement traditional treatments, they should be pursued under the guidance of qualified health professionals. The synergy of conventional and natural therapies can provide a comprehensive approach to cancer care, aiming not just to treat the disease but to improve the overall well-being of the patient.

CHAPTER 10: NATURAL REMEDIES FOR HEART DISEASE

Heart disease remains one of the leading causes of mortality globally, but there's a growing interest in how natural remedies and lifestyle changes can support heart health. The heart, a remarkable organ, has its rhythm, vital for maintaining life. When we talk about heart health, we're not just focusing on preventing or managing heart disease; we're also talking about nurturing this vital rhythm and ensuring our heart functions optimally.

The Heart's Natural Rhythm

The heart's rhythm is more than just its beat. It involves complex interactions between electrical impulses, muscle function, and blood flow. A healthy rhythm ensures that blood is efficiently pumped throughout the body, delivering essential nutrients and oxygen to various organs. When this rhythm is disrupted, it can lead to various heart conditions.

Maintaining a natural and healthy heart rhythm involves a blend of good nutrition, regular exercise, stress management, and avoiding harmful habits like smoking and excessive alcohol consumption. It's about creating a balance in our lifestyles that supports our heart's natural function.

Lifestyle Interventions for Heart Health

1. **Diet:** A heart-healthy diet is rich in fruits, vegetables, whole grains, lean proteins, and healthy fats. Foods like salmon, rich in omega-3 fatty acids, and berries, loaded with antioxidants, are particularly beneficial. Minimizing intake of processed foods, salt, and unhealthy fats is also crucial.

2. **Exercise:** Regular physical activity is key. It doesn't have to be intense; even moderate activities like brisk walking or cycling can strengthen the heart. Aim for at least 150 minutes of moderate aerobic exercise per week.

3. **Stress Management:** Chronic stress can negatively impact heart health. Practices like yoga, meditation, and deep breathing exercises can help manage stress levels.

4. **Sleep:** Adequate and quality sleep is essential. Poor sleep patterns have been linked to higher risks of heart disease.

Supplements for Cardiovascular Support

Alongside lifestyle changes, certain supplements may offer additional support:

1. **Omega-3 Fatty Acids:** Found in fish oil, they help reduce triglycerides, lower blood pressure slightly, and reduce blood clotting.

2. **Coenzyme Q10 (CoQ10):** This naturally occurring antioxidant may help with heart muscle function and blood pressure.

3. **Magnesium:** Essential for heart rhythm, it helps regulate blood pressure and is vital for muscle function.

4. **Garlic:** Known for its cholesterol-lowering and blood pressure-reducing properties.

5. **Green Tea Extract:** Rich in antioxidants, it's been linked to improved heart health, though moderation is key due to its caffeine content.

Remember, while these natural remedies can support heart health, they're not replacements for medical treatment in the case of existing heart conditions. Always consult with a healthcare professional before starting any new supplement, especially if you have health concerns or are on medication.

In summary, taking care of your heart involves a holistic approach. A balanced diet, regular exercise, managing stress, getting quality sleep, and possibly including some heart-supporting supplements, are all strategies that work in harmony to keep your heart healthy. By understanding and respecting our heart's natural rhythm, we can take significant steps toward preventing heart disease and maintaining overall health.

CHAPTER 11: NATURAL REMEDIES FOR DIABETES

Diabetes, a condition characterized by high blood sugar levels, can be a challenging journey for many. It's not just about managing numbers; it's about a lifestyle overhaul. Thankfully, nature has provided us with numerous tools to help in this battle. We'll explore how balancing blood sugar naturally, using supplements, and making lifestyle changes can be effective strategies for managing diabetes.

The Basics of Blood Sugar Control

Blood sugar control is the cornerstone of managing diabetes. The goal here is to maintain a steady glucose level, avoiding spikes and drops. It starts with understanding the glycemic index (GI) of foods. Foods with a low GI are slower to raise blood sugar levels. Incorporating these into your diet is key. Think fiber-rich foods like whole grains, legumes, and plenty of vegetables. They not only slow down glucose absorption but also keep you full, reducing the urge to snack on sugary treats.

Regular monitoring is crucial. Keeping track of blood sugar levels helps in understanding how different foods and activities affect your body. This insight allows for more informed choices in both diet and lifestyle.

Natural Supplements for Diabetes

Nature's pharmacy offers several options that can support blood sugar control:

- **Cinnamon**: More than just a spice, cinnamon has been shown to have a positive effect on blood sugar levels. It can improve insulin sensitivity, making your body's cells better at using the available sugar.

- **Bitter Melon**: This might not be your favorite vegetable, but its glucose-lowering effect is worth noting. Bitter melon contains compounds that act like insulin, helping lower blood sugar levels.

- **Magnesium**: Low magnesium levels are common in people with diabetes. Supplementing with magnesium can improve insulin sensitivity and may help prevent diabetes-related complications.

- **Omega-3 Fatty Acids**: Found in fish oil and flaxseeds, these fats are not only good for the heart but also may help in regulating blood sugar levels.

Remember, supplements should complement, not replace, standard diabetes treatments. Always consult with a healthcare provider before starting any new supplement.

Lifestyle Changes to Manage Diabetes

Lifestyle modifications are perhaps the most powerful tool in the diabetes management kit. Here are some key changes:

- **Exercise**: Regular physical activity is a must. It helps in using up the glucose in your blood for energy and muscle building, lowering blood sugar levels. A mix of cardio, strength training, and flexibility exercises is ideal.

- **Weight Management**: If you're overweight, losing even a small amount of weight can have a significant impact on your blood sugar control.

- **Stress Management**: Stress can wreak havoc on blood sugar levels. Practices like yoga, meditation, or even simple deep breathing exercises can be immensely beneficial.

- **Sleep Quality**: Poor sleep can affect blood sugar levels and insulin sensitivity. Aim for 7-8 hours of quality sleep each night.

- **Smoking and Alcohol**: Both can affect blood sugar levels. Quitting smoking and moderating alcohol intake can improve diabetes control.

In conclusion, managing diabetes naturally involves a comprehensive approach encompassing diet, supplements, and lifestyle changes. It's about creating a balance, listening to your body, and making adjustments that work for you. With the right strategies, diabetes can be managed effectively, allowing for a healthy, fulfilling life.

CHAPTER 12: PREVENTION STRATEGIES

When it comes to managing health, the adage "prevention is better than cure" is more relevant than ever. In a world where chronic diseases like cancer, heart disease, and diabetes are prevalent, taking proactive steps to prevent these conditions is crucial. This chapter will delve into effective prevention strategies that prioritize maintaining health and well-being before the onset of disease. We'll explore how to preemptively tackle health issues, the importance of early detection, and natural remedies that can strengthen your immune system.

Preventing Disease Before It Starts

The first line of defense in disease prevention is lifestyle. Your daily habits significantly influence your risk of developing various health conditions. Here's how you can create a lifestyle conducive to preventing diseases:

1. **Nutrition**: Opt for a diet rich in fruits, vegetables, whole grains, and lean proteins. These foods are loaded with essential nutrients that support overall health and help ward off diseases.

2. **Physical Activity**: Regular exercise is key. It doesn't have to be rigorous; even moderate activities like brisk walking or cycling can have substantial health benefits.

3. **Stress Management**: Chronic stress can take a toll on your body, making it susceptible to illnesses. Techniques such as meditation, yoga, and deep breathing can help manage stress effectively.

4. **Adequate Sleep**: Quality sleep is vital. It helps in the repair and rejuvenation of your body. Aim for 7-8 hours of uninterrupted sleep each night.

5. **Avoiding Harmful Substances**: Reducing alcohol consumption and quitting smoking are critical steps in disease prevention.

Early Detection and Natural Remedies

Detecting a health issue early can make a significant difference in treatment and outcomes. Regular health check-ups and screenings are vital, especially if you have a family history of certain diseases. Natural remedies can complement these efforts:

1. **Herbal Supplements**: Certain herbs like turmeric, ginger, and garlic are known for

their anti-inflammatory and antioxidant properties.

2. **Functional Foods**: Incorporate foods like blueberries, nuts, and green tea, which are renowned for their health-promoting properties.

3. **Mind-Body Practices**: Techniques such as Tai Chi and Qi Gong promote mental and physical well-being, which can help in early detection by increasing body awareness.

Building a Resilient Immune System

A strong immune system is your best defense against diseases. Here's how you can bolster it:

1. **Nutrient-Rich Diet**: A diet high in vitamins and minerals, particularly vitamin C, vitamin D, zinc, and selenium, is crucial for a robust immune system.

2. **Regular Exercise**: This not only keeps you fit but also enhances your immune response.

3. **Adequate Sleep and Hydration**: Never underestimate the power of good sleep and staying hydrated in keeping your immune system functioning optimally.

4. **Probiotics**: These beneficial bacteria play a key role in gut health, which is closely linked to immune function.

5. **Reducing Stress**: Chronic stress weakens the immune system, so managing stress is key to maintaining good health.

Prevention strategies are all about taking charge of your health proactively. By incorporating healthy lifestyle choices, staying vigilant through early detection, and nurturing your immune system, you're setting the foundation for a healthier, disease-free life. Remember, each small step you take can have a significant impact on your overall well-being.

CHAPTER 13: CREATING YOUR OWN NATURAL REMEDY PLAN

Creating your own natural remedy plan is a journey toward personal wellness, blending age-old wisdom with a modern understanding of health. It's about taking control of your health narrative and finding natural ways to support your body's healing process.

Assessing Your Health Status

The first step in this journey is to assess your current health status. It's like taking a snapshot of where you are right now. This involves looking at various aspects:

1. **Medical History**: A thorough review of your past and current medical conditions, surgeries, and treatments.

2. **Lifestyle Evaluation**: Observing your daily habits, diet, exercise routine, sleep patterns, and stress levels.

3. **Symptom Check**: Noting any specific symptoms you experience regularly, even if they seem minor.

4. **Professional Health Assessments**: If possible, getting a professional health

assessment, including blood tests, can provide a detailed overview of your health status.

The idea is to gather as much information as possible. This will serve as the foundation upon which your natural remedy plan is built.

Setting Personal Health Goals

Next, let's talk about setting health goals. This isn't about setting lofty, unachievable targets but about identifying realistic, incremental steps to improve your health. Goals can be diverse, such as:

- Improving energy levels
- Reducing the symptoms of a specific condition
- Achieving a balanced diet
- Enhancing mental wellbeing
- Building physical strength or endurance

The key is to make these goals specific, measurable, achievable, relevant, and time-bound (SMART). For instance, instead of saying "I want to be healthier," you might say, "I aim to walk 30 minutes daily for the next three months to improve cardiovascular health."

Developing a Personalized Remedy Plan

Now, the most action-oriented part: developing your remedy plan. This is where you translate your assessment and goals into a concrete plan. Here are the steps to consider:

1. **Dietary Adjustments**: Based on your health assessment, identify what dietary changes could benefit you. This might include incorporating more anti-inflammatory foods or reducing sugar intake.

2. **Herbal Supplements**: Research and identify herbs that might be beneficial for your specific health concerns. Remember, it's crucial to consult with a healthcare provider before starting any new supplement, especially if you have existing health conditions or are on medication.

3. **Lifestyle Changes**: Incorporate lifestyle modifications that align with your goals. This could be adopting a new exercise routine, improving sleep hygiene, or practicing stress-reduction techniques like meditation or yoga.

4. **Tracking Progress**: Set up a system to monitor your progress. This could be a

health journal, an app, or regular check-ins with a health professional.

5. **Adjusting As Needed**: Be prepared to adjust your plan as you go. Your body will give you feedback, and it's important to listen and adapt accordingly.

In creating this plan, remember that the journey is uniquely yours. What works for one person may not work for another, and that's perfectly okay. The aim is to find what resonates with your body and lifestyle. Always consult healthcare professionals when making significant changes to your health regimen, especially if you have existing health conditions. With patience, persistence, and a bit of experimentation, you can craft a natural remedy plan that supports your journey to better health.

HEALTHY RECIPES THAT FIGHT OFF DISEASES

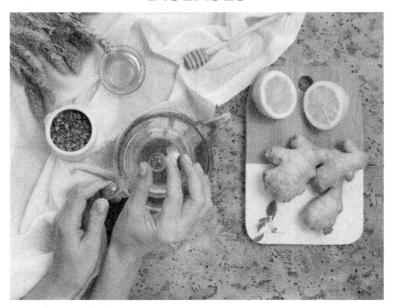

Breakfast Recipes:

Berry Blast Smoothie

Preparation Time: 5 minutes | Cooking Time: 0 minutes| Total Time: 5 minutes| Number of Servings: 2

Ingredients:

- 1 cup mixed berries (blueberries, strawberries, raspberries)
- 1 banana
- 1 cup spinach
- 1 tablespoon flaxseeds
- 1 cup Greek yogurt

- 1 cup water

Directions:

- Blend all the ingredients until smooth.
- Pour into glasses and enjoy.

Nutrition Per Serving: Calories: 250 | Protein: 12g | Carbohydrates: 40g | Fiber: 8g | Fat: 5g

Turmeric Scramble

Preparation Time: 10 minutes | Cooking Time: 10 minutes | Total Time: 20 minutes | Number of Servings: 2

Ingredients:

- 4 large eggs
- 1/2 teaspoon turmeric
- 1 cup broccoli florets
- 1 cup sliced mushrooms
- Salt and pepper to taste

Directions:

- In a bowl, beat the eggs and add turmeric, salt, and pepper.
- Heat a non-stick pan, add broccoli and mushrooms, and sauté until tender.
- Pour the egg mixture over the veggies and scramble until cooked.
- Serve hot.

Nutrition Per Serving: Calories: 220 | Protein: 16g | Carbohydrates: 6g | Fiber: 3g | Fat: 15g

Chia Seed Pudding

Preparation Time: 5 minutes (plus overnight soaking)| Cooking Time: 0 minutes| Total Time: 5 minutes (plus overnight soaking)| Number of Servings: 2

Ingredients:
- 1/4 cup chia seeds
- 1 cup almond milk
- 1 teaspoon honey
- 1/2 teaspoon vanilla extract
- 1/2 cup mixed berries

Directions:

- In a jar, combine chia seeds, almond milk, honey, and vanilla extract.
- Stir well, cover, and refrigerate overnight.
- In the morning, top with mixed berries and enjoy.

Nutrition Per Serving: Calories: 170 | Protein: 4g | Carbohydrates: 20g | Fiber: 11g | Fat: 9g

Avocado Toast

Preparation Time: 5 minutes| Cooking Time: 0 minutes| Total Time: 5 minutes| Number of Servings: 2

Ingredients:

- 2 slices of whole-grain bread
- 1 ripe avocado
- 1 tomato, sliced

- 1 tablespoon olive oil

Directions:

- Toast the bread until crispy.
- Mash the avocado and spread it on the toast.
- Top with tomato slices, drizzle with olive oil and add a pinch of salt.

Nutrition Per Serving: Calories: 250 | Protein: 5g | Carbohydrates: 20g | Fiber: 7g | Fat: 18g

Oatmeal Power Bowl

Preparation Time: 5 minutes | Cooking Time: 5 minutes | Total Time: 10 minutes | Number of Servings: 2

Ingredients:

- 1 cup rolled oats
- 1 teaspoon cinnamon
- 1/4 cup chopped walnuts
- 1 apple, sliced
- 2 cups water

Directions:

- In a saucepan, combine oats, cinnamon, walnuts, and water.
- Cook over medium heat, stirring, until creamy.
- Serve with sliced apples on top.

Nutrition Per Serving: Calories: 300 | Protein: 8g | Carbohydrates: 50g | Fiber: 10g | Fat: 10g

Green Tea and Chia Seed Smoothie

Preparation Time: 5 minutes | Cooking Time: 0 minutes | Total Time: 5 minutes | Number of Servings: 2

Ingredients:

- 2 cups brewed green tea, cooled
- 2 tablespoons chia seeds
- 1 cup fresh pineapple chunks
- 1 small cucumber, peeled and chopped

Directions:

- Blend green tea, chia seeds, pineapple, and cucumber until smooth.
- Pour into glasses and enjoy this antioxidant-rich smoothie.

Nutrition Per Serving: Calories: 80 | Protein: 2g | Carbohydrates: 16g | Fiber: 6g | Fat: 2g

Sweet Potato and Spinach Frittata

Preparation Time: 10 minutes | Cooking Time: 20 minutes | Total Time: 30 minutes | Number of Servings: 4

Ingredients:

- 2 sweet potatoes, peeled and sliced
- 2 cups fresh spinach
- 8 eggs

- 1/2 cup feta cheese
- Salt and pepper to taste

Directions*:*

- Preheat the oven to 350°F (175°C).
- Steam the sweet potato slices until tender.
- In a bowl, whisk eggs, add spinach, feta, sweet potatoes, salt, and pepper.
- Pour the mixture into a greased ovenproof skillet and bake for 20 minutes or until set.

Nutrition Per Serving: Calories: 250 | Protein: 13g | Carbohydrates: 14g | Fiber: 2g | Fat: 15g

Almond Butter and Banana Pancakes

Preparation Time: 10 minutes| Cooking Time: 10 minutes| Total Time: 20 minutes| Number of Servings: 2

Ingredients*:*

- 1 cup almond butter
- 2 ripe bananas
- 2 eggs
- 1 teaspoon baking powder

Directions*:*

- In a blender, combine almond butter, bananas, eggs, and baking powder.
- Heat a non-stick skillet and pour small portions of the batter to make pancakes.

- Cook until bubbles form on top, then flip and cook the other side.

Nutrition Per Serving: Calories: 400 | Protein: 15g | Carbohydrates: 20g | Fiber: 5g | Fat: 30g

Spinach and Mushroom Omelette

Preparation Time: 10 minutes| Cooking Time: 10 minutes| Total Time: 20 minutes| Number of Servings: 2

Ingredients:

- 4 large eggs
- 1 cup fresh spinach
- 1 cup sliced mushrooms
- 1/4 cup grated Parmesan cheese
- Salt and pepper to taste

Directions:

- In a bowl, beat the eggs, and add salt, pepper, and Parmesan cheese.
- Heat a non-stick skillet, add spinach and mushrooms, and sauté until wilted.
- Pour the egg mixture over the veggies and cook until set.

Nutrition Per Serving: Calories: 200 | Protein: 14g | Carbohydrates: 4g | Fiber: 2g | Fat: 15g

Golden Milk Overnight Oats

Preparation Time: 10 minutes (plus overnight soaking)| Cooking Time: 0 minutes | Total Time: 10

minutes (plus overnight soaking)| Number of Servings: 2

Ingredients:

- 1 cup rolled oats
- 1 teaspoon turmeric
- 1/2 teaspoon cinnamon
- 1/4 cup honey
- 1 1/2 cups almond milk

Directions:

- In a jar, combine oats, turmeric, cinnamon, honey, and almond milk.
- Stir well, cover, and refrigerate overnight.
- In the morning, enjoy this anti-inflammatory and energizing breakfast.

Nutrition Per Serving: Calories: 300 | Protein: 7g | Carbohydrates: 50g | Fiber: 7g | Fat: 8g

Lunch Recipes:

Quinoa and Black Bean Salad

Preparation Time: 15 minutes| Cooking Time: 15 minutes| Total Time: 30 minutes| Number of Servings: 4

Ingredients*:*

- 1 cup quinoa, cooked
- 1 can (15 oz) black beans, drained and rinsed
- 1 cup corn kernels (fresh or frozen)
- 1 red bell pepper, diced
- 1/4 cup fresh cilantro, chopped
- Lime vinaigrette (lime juice, olive oil, and a touch of honey)

Directions*:*

- In a large bowl, combine quinoa, black beans, corn, bell pepper, and cilantro.
- Drizzle with lime vinaigrette and toss to combine.

Nutrition Per Serving: Calories: 350 | Protein: 11g | Carbohydrates: 60g | Fiber: 12g | Fat: 8g

Tuna and White Bean Salad

Preparation Time: 10 minutes| Cooking Time: 0 minutes| Total Time: 10 minutes| Number of Servings: 2

Ingredients*:*

- 2 cans (5 oz each) of tuna in water, drained
- 1 can (15 oz) white beans, drained and rinsed
- 1/2 red onion, finely chopped
- 2 tablespoons fresh parsley, chopped
- Lemon and olive oil dressing

Directions*:*

- In a large bowl, combine tuna, white beans, red onion, and parsley.
- Drizzle with lemon and olive oil dressing and mix well.

Nutrition Per Serving: Calories: 350 | Protein: 40g | Carbohydrates: 35g | Fiber: 9g | Fat: 8g

Roasted Vegetable and Quinoa Bowl

Preparation Time: 15 minutes| Cooking Time: 25 minutes| Total Time: 40 minutes| Number of Servings: 2

Ingredients*:*

- 1 cup quinoa, cooked
- Assorted roasted vegetables (e.g., sweet potatoes, bell peppers, zucchini)
- 1/4 cup hummus
- 2 tablespoons tahini dressing

Directions*:*

- Roast your choice of vegetables in the oven until tender.

- In a bowl, assemble quinoa, and roasted vegetables, and top with hummus and tahini dressing.

Nutrition Per Serving: Calories: 400 | Protein: 12g | Carbohydrates: 60g | Fiber: 10g | Fat: 14g

Lentil and Spinach Soup

Preparation Time: 10 minutes | Cooking Time: 30 minutes | Total Time: 40 minutes | Number of Servings: 4

Ingredients:

- 1 cup green or brown lentils, rinsed
- 1 onion, chopped
- 2 carrots, chopped
- 2 celery stalks, chopped
- 4 cups vegetable broth
- 2 cups fresh spinach

Directions:

- In a pot, sauté onion, carrots, and celery until soft.
- Add lentils and vegetable broth, bring to a boil, and simmer until lentils are tender.
- Stir in fresh spinach until wilted.

Nutrition Per Serving: Calories: 250 | Protein: 15g | Carbohydrates: 40g | Fiber: 15g | Fat: 2g

Grilled Chicken and Quinoa Salad

Preparation Time: 20 minutes| Cooking Time: 15 minutes| Total Time: 35 minutes| Number of Servings: 4

Ingredients*:*

- 2 boneless, skinless chicken breasts
- 1 cup quinoa, cooked
- 1 cucumber, diced
- 1 cup cherry tomatoes, halved
- 1/4 cup fresh basil, chopped
- Balsamic vinaigrette dressing

Directions*:*

- Grill the chicken until cooked through, then slice it.
- In a bowl, combine quinoa, cucumber, cherry tomatoes, and basil.
- Drizzle with balsamic vinaigrette and top with grilled chicken.

Nutrition Per Serving: Calories: 350 | Protein: 30g | Carbohydrates: 40g | Fiber: 5g | Fat: 8g

Mediterranean Chickpea Salad

Preparation Time: 15 minutes| Cooking Time: 0 minutes| Total Time: 15 minutes| Number of Servings: 4

Ingredients*:*

- 2 cans (15 oz each) chickpeas, drained and rinsed
- 1 cucumber, diced
- 1 cup cherry tomatoes, halved
- 1/2 red onion, finely chopped
- Feta cheese (optional)
- Olive oil and lemon juice dressing

Directions:

- In a large bowl, combine chickpeas, cucumber, cherry tomatoes, and red onion.
- Drizzle with olive oil and lemon juice dressing.
- Add crumbled feta cheese if desired.

Nutrition Per Serving: Calories: 300 | Protein: 12g | Carbohydrates: 45g | Fiber: 10g | Fat: 10g

Spinach and Quinoa Stuffed Bell Peppers

Preparation Time: 15 minutes| Cooking Time: 45 minutes| Total Time: 1 hour| Number of Servings: 4

Ingredients:

- 4 bell peppers, tops removed and seeds removed
- 1 cup quinoa, cooked
- 2 cups fresh spinach
- 1 can (15 oz) diced tomatoes
- 1/2 cup grated Parmesan cheese

Directions:

- Preheat the oven to 375°F (190°C).
- In a bowl, mix cooked quinoa, fresh spinach, diced tomatoes, and Parmesan cheese.
- Stuff each bell pepper with the quinoa mixture.
- Bake for 30-40 minutes or until peppers are tender.

Nutrition Per Serving: Calories: 250 | Protein: 10g | Carbohydrates: 40g | Fiber: 7g | Fat: 6g

Asian-Inspired Salmon Salad

Preparation Time: 20 minutes | Cooking Time: 10 minutes | Total Time: 30 minutes | Number of Servings: 2

Ingredients*:*

- 2 salmon fillets
- 2 cups mixed greens
- 1/2 cup edamame beans
- 1/4 cup sliced almonds
- Soy-ginger dressing

Directions*:*

- Grill or pan-sear the salmon until cooked.
- In a bowl, combine mixed greens, edamame beans, and sliced almonds.
- Top with cooked salmon and drizzle with soy-ginger dressing.

Nutrition Per Serving: Calories: 350 | Protein: 25g | Carbohydrates: 14g | Fiber: 5g | Fat: 20g

Zucchini Noodles with Pesto

Preparation Time: 15 minutes| Cooking Time: 10 minutes| Total Time: 25 minutes| Number of Servings: 2

Ingredients*:*

- 2 medium zucchinis, spiralized into noodles
- 1/2 cup homemade basil and walnut pesto
- 1 cup cherry tomatoes, halved
- Grated Parmesan cheese (optional)

Directions:

- In a pan, sauté zucchini noodles until tender.
- Toss the cooked noodles with homemade pesto.
- Top with cherry tomatoes and grated Parmesan if desired.

Nutrition Per Serving: Calories: 280 | Protein: 5g | Carbohydrates: 12g | Fiber: 3g | Fat: 23g

Lentil and Vegetable Stir-Fry

Preparation Time: 20 minutes| Cooking Time: 15 minutes| Total Time: 35 minutes| Number of Servings: 4

Ingredients*:*

- 1 cup brown lentils, cooked
- Mixed stir-fry vegetables (e.g., broccoli, bell peppers, snap peas)
- Stir-fry sauce (soy sauce, ginger, and garlic)
- Sesame seeds for garnish

Directions*:*

- In a pan, stir-fry the mixed vegetables until tender-crisp.
- Add cooked brown lentils and stir-fry sauce.
- Garnish with sesame seeds.

Nutrition Per Serving: Calories: 280 | Protein: 15g | Carbohydrates: 40g | Fiber: 12g | Fat: 3g

Dinner Recipes:

Turmeric Lentil Soup

Preparation Time: 15 minutes| Cooking Time: 30 minutes| Total Time: 45 minutes| Number of Servings: 4

Ingredients:

- 1 cup red lentils
- 1 onion, chopped
- 2 carrots, chopped
- 2 teaspoons turmeric
- 4 cups vegetable broth
- Juice of 1 lemon

Directions:

- In a large pot, sauté onions and carrots until soft.
- Add red lentils, turmeric, and vegetable broth. Simmer until lentils are tender.
- Stir in lemon juice before serving.

Nutrition Per Serving: Calories: 280 | Protein: 15g | Carbohydrates: 40g | Fiber: 10g | Fat: 2g

Garlic and Lemon Shrimp

Preparation Time: 10 minutes| Cooking Time: 10 minutes| Total Time: 20 minutes | Number of Servings: 2

Ingredients:

- large shrimp peeled and deveined

- 4 cloves garlic, minced
- Juice of 1 lemon
- 2 tablespoons olive oil

Directions*:*

- In a pan, heat olive oil and sauté garlic until fragrant.
- Add shrimp and cook until pink and opaque.
- Drizzle with lemon juice before serving.

Nutrition Per Serving: Calories: 220 | Protein: 25g | Carbohydrates: 4g | Fiber: 0g | Fat: 13g

Broccoli and Mushroom Stir-Fry

Preparation Time: 15 minutes| Cooking Time: 15 minutes| Total Time: 30 minutes| Number of Servings: 4

Ingredients*:*

- 1 pound broccoli florets
- 2 cups sliced mushrooms
- 1 block tofu, cubed
- Stir-fry sauce (soy sauce, ginger, and garlic)
- Brown rice (optional)

Directions*:*

- In a wok or large pan, stir-fry broccoli and mushrooms until tender-crisp.
- Add cubed tofu and stir-fry sauce.
- Serve over brown rice if desired.

Nutrition Per Serving: Calories: 220 | Protein: 15g | Carbohydrates: 15g | Fiber: 6g | Fat: 10g

Cauliflower Rice Pilaf

Preparation Time: 15 minutes| Cooking Time: 15 minutes| Total Time: 30 minutes| Number of Servings: 4

Ingredients*:*

- 1 head of cauliflower, grated into rice-like pieces
- 1 cup mixed vegetables (e.g., peas, carrots, corn)
- 1/4 cup chopped almonds
- 1 teaspoon cumin

Directions*:*

- In a large pan, sauté cauliflower "rice" and mixed vegetables until heated through.
- Stir in chopped almonds and cumin.

Nutrition Per Serving: Calories: 150 | Protein: 5g | Carbohydrates: 18g | Fiber: 6g | Fat: 7g

Spaghetti Squash with Pesto

Preparation Time: 15 minutes| Cooking Time: 40 minutes| Total Time: 55 minutes| Number of Servings: 2

Ingredients*:*

- 1 spaghetti squash, halved and seeds removed

- Homemade basil and walnut pesto
- Grated Parmesan cheese (optional)

Directions*:*

- Roast the spaghetti squash in the oven until the flesh is tender and shreds like spaghetti.
- Toss with homemade pesto.
- Top with grated Parmesan cheese if desired.

Nutrition Per Serving: Calories: 250 | Protein: 5g | Carbohydrates: 30g | Fiber: 5g | Fat: 13g

Baked Salmon with Quinoa and Asparagus

Preparation Time: 15 minutes| Cooking Time: 25 minutes| Total Time: 40 minutes| Number of Servings: 4

Ingredients*:*

- 4 salmon fillets
- 1 cup quinoa, cooked
- 1 bunch asparagus, trimmed
- Lemon-dill sauce

Directions*:*

- Preheat the oven to 375°F (190°C).
- Place salmon fillets on a baking sheet and surround with asparagus.
- Bake until salmon flakes easily and asparagus is tender.

- Serve with cooked quinoa and drizzle with lemon-dill sauce.

Nutrition Per Serving: Calories: 350 | Protein: 30g | Carbohydrates: 30g | Fiber: 7g | Fat: 12g

Quinoa-Stuffed Portobello Mushrooms

Preparation Time: 20 minutes| Cooking Time: 25 minutes| Total Time: 45 minutes| Number of Servings: 4

Ingredients*:*

- 4 large Portobello mushrooms, stems removed
- 1 cup quinoa, cooked
- 1 cup spinach, chopped
- 1/4 cup sundried tomatoes, chopped
- Feta cheese (optional)

Directions*:*

- Preheat the oven to 375°F (190°C).
- Place Portobello mushrooms on a baking sheet and roast for 10 minutes.
- In a bowl, mix cooked quinoa, chopped spinach, and sundried tomatoes.
- Stuff the mushrooms with the quinoa mixture and return to the oven for 15 minutes.
- Top with crumbled feta cheese if desired.

Nutrition Per Serving: Calories: 250 | Protein: 10g | Carbohydrates: 40g | Fiber: 7g | Fat: 6g

Vegetable Curry with Chickpeas

Preparation Time: 15 minutes| Cooking Time: 30 minutes| Total Time: 45 minutes| Number of Servings: 4

Ingredients*:*

- 2 cups mixed vegetables (e.g., cauliflower, bell peppers, peas)
- 1 can (15 oz) chickpeas, drained and rinsed
- 1 can (14 oz) coconut milk
- 2 tablespoons curry paste

Directions*:*

- In a large pot, sauté mixed vegetables and curry paste until fragrant.
- Add chickpeas and coconut milk.
- Simmer until the vegetables are tender.

Nutrition Per Serving: Calories: 350 | Protein: 10g | Carbohydrates: 40g | Fiber: 8g | Fat: 15g

Turmeric-Ginger Chicken Stir-Fry

Preparation Time: 20 minutes| Cooking Time: 15 minutes| Total Time: 35 minutes| Number of Servings: 4

Ingredients*:*

- 2 boneless, skinless chicken breasts, cubed
- 2 teaspoons turmeric

- 1 tablespoon grated ginger
- Mixed stir-fry vegetables
- Soy sauce

Directions*:*

- In a wok or large pan, stir-fry chicken with turmeric and ginger until cooked through.
- Add mixed stir-fry vegetables and soy sauce.
- Cook until vegetables are tender.

Nutrition Per Serving: Calories: 280 | Protein: 30g | Carbohydrates: 20g | Fiber: 6g | Fat: 8g

Stuffed Bell Peppers with Turkey and Quinoa

Preparation Time: 20 minutes| Cooking Time: 40 minutes| Total Time: 1 hour| Number of Servings: 4

Ingredients*:*

- 4 bell peppers, tops removed and seeds removed
- 1 cup ground turkey
- 1 cup cooked quinoa
- 1 can (14 oz) diced tomatoes
- 1/2 cup shredded mozzarella cheese

Directions*:*

- Preheat the oven to 375°F (190°C).
- In a pan, cook ground turkey until browned.

- In a bowl, combine cooked turkey, quinoa, diced tomatoes, and 1/4 cup of mozzarella cheese.
- Stuff each bell pepper with the mixture.
- Bake for 30-40 minutes until the peppers are tender and the cheese is bubbly.

Nutrition Per Serving: Calories: 300 | Protein: 20g | Carbohydrates: 30g | Fiber: 5g | Fat: 12g

Snack Recipes:

Homemade Hummus with Veggie Sticks

Preparation Time: 10 minutes| Cooking Time: 0 minutes| Total Time: 10 minutes| Number of Servings: 4

Ingredients*:*

- 1 can (15 oz) chickpeas, drained and rinsed
- 2 tablespoons tahini
- 2 cloves garlic
- Juice of 1 lemon
- Carrot, cucumber, and bell pepper sticks for dipping

Directions*:*

- In a food processor, blend chickpeas, tahini, garlic, and lemon juice until smooth.
- Serve with an assortment of veggie sticks for dipping.

Nutrition Per Serving: Calories: 180 | Protein: 6g | Carbohydrates: 20g | Fiber: 5g | Fat: 8g

Almond and Berry Trail Mix

Preparation Time: 5 minutes| Cooking Time: 0 minutes| Total Time: 5 minutes| Number of Servings: 4

Ingredients*:*

- 1 cup raw almonds
- 1/2 cup dried cranberries

- 1/2 cup dried blueberries
- 1/4 cup dark chocolate chips

Directions*:*

- Mix almonds, dried cranberries, dried blueberries, and dark chocolate chips.
- Portion into snack-sized bags for a quick grab-and-go option.

Nutrition Per Serving: Calories: 250 | Protein: 6g | Carbohydrates: 30g | Fiber: 5g | Fat: 14g

Greek Yogurt Parfait

Preparation Time: 5 minutes| Cooking Time: 0 minutes| Total Time: 5 minutes| Number of Servings: 2

Ingredients*:*

- 2 cups Greek yogurt
- 1/2 cup granola
- 1 cup mixed berries (blueberries, strawberries, raspberries)
- Honey for drizzling

Directions*:*

- In serving glasses, layer Greek yogurt, granola, mixed berries, and drizzle with honey.
- Repeat the layers.
- Enjoy this protein-packed snack.

Nutrition Per Serving: Calories: 300 | Protein: 15g | Carbohydrates: 40g | Fiber: 5g | Fat: 10g

Cucumber and Hummus Bites

Preparation Time: 10 minutes| Cooking Time: 0 minutes| Total Time: 10 minutes| Number of Servings: 4

Ingredients*:*

- 2 large cucumbers, sliced into rounds
- 1/2 cup hummus
- Cherry tomatoes for garnish

Directions*:*

- Place cucumber slices on a platter.
- Add a dollop of hummus to each cucumber round.
- Garnish with halved cherry tomatoes.

Nutrition Per Serving: Calories: 90 | Protein: 4g | Carbohydrates: 12g | Fiber: 4g | Fat: 3g

Chia Seed Energy Bars

Preparation Time: 20 minutes| Cooking Time: 0 minutes| Total Time: 20 minutes| Number of Servings: 8

Ingredients*:*

- 1/2 cup chia seeds
- 1/2 cup rolled oats
- 1/2 cup almond butter
- 1/4 cup honey

- 1/4 cup dried apricots, chopped

Directions*:*

- In a bowl, mix chia seeds, rolled oats, almond butter, honey, and dried apricots.
- Press the mixture into a lined pan.
- Refrigerate until firm, then cut into bars.

Nutrition Per Serving: Calories: 220 | Protein: 5g | Carbohydrates: 20g | Fiber: 6g | Fat: 12g

Avocado and Salsa Rice Cakes

Preparation Time: 5 minutes| Cooking Time: 0 minutes| Total Time: 5 minutes| Number of Servings: 2

Ingredients*:*

- 2 rice cakes
- 1 ripe avocado, mashed
- Salsa for topping

Directions*:*

- Spread mashed avocado evenly on rice cakes.
- Top with salsa for a burst of flavor and healthy fats.

Nutrition Per Serving: Calories: 180 | Protein: 3g | Carbohydrates: 15g | Fiber: 7g | Fat: 13g

Mixed Nuts and Dried Fruit

Preparation Time: 5 minutes| Cooking Time: 0 minutes| Total Time: 5 minutes| Number of Servings: 4

Ingredients:

- 1 cup mixed unsalted nuts (e.g., almonds, walnuts, cashews)
- 1/2 cup mixed dried fruit (e.g., raisins, apricots, cranberries)

Directions:

- Mix nuts and dried fruit in a bowl.
- Portion into snack-sized bags for a quick energy boost.

Nutrition Per Serving: Calories: 250 | Protein: 6g | Carbohydrates: 25g | Fiber: 4g | Fat: 15g

Edamame with Sea Salt

Preparation Time: 10 minutes| Cooking Time: 5 minutes| Total Time: 15 minutes| Number of Servings: 4

Ingredients:

- 2 cups frozen edamame
- Sea salt for seasoning

Directions:

- Cook edamame according to package instructions.

- Season with sea salt for a simple and satisfying snack.

Nutrition Per Serving: Calories: 100 | Protein: 8g | Carbohydrates: 8g | Fiber: 4g | Fat: 4g

Roasted Red Pepper and Walnut Dip

Preparation Time: 15 minutes| Cooking Time: 10 minutes| Total Time: 25 minutes| Number of Servings: 6

Ingredients:

- 2 red bell peppers
- 1/2 cup walnuts
- 2 cloves garlic
- 2 tablespoons olive oil

Directions:

- Roast red bell peppers until charred, then peel and remove seeds.
- In a food processor, blend roasted peppers, walnuts, garlic, and olive oil.
- Serve as a dip with whole-grain crackers or vegetable sticks.

Nutrition Per Serving: Calories: 140 | Protein: 3g | Carbohydrates: 5g | Fiber: 2g | Fat: 12g

Greek Cucumber Cups

Preparation Time: 15 minutes| Cooking Time: 0 minutes| Total Time: 15 minutes| Number of Servings: 4

Ingredients*:*

- 2 cucumbers
- 1 cup Greek yogurt
- 1/2 cup cherry tomatoes, chopped
- Fresh dill for garnish

Directions*:*

- Cut cucumbers into thick slices and scoop out the centers to create cups.
- Fill the cucumber cups with Greek yogurt.
- Top with chopped cherry tomatoes and fresh dill.

Nutrition Per Serving: Calories: 80 | Protein: 6g | Carbohydrates: 6g | Fiber: 1g | Fat: 4g

Dessert Recipes:

Berry and Chia Seed Pudding

Preparation Time: 10 minutes | Cooking Time: 0 minutes | Total Time: 4 hours (for chilling) | Number of Servings: 4

Ingredients:

- 1 cup mixed berries (strawberries, blueberries, raspberries)
- 1/4 cup chia seeds
- 2 cups unsweetened almond milk
- 2 tablespoons honey or maple syrup (optional)

Directions:

- In a bowl, mix chia seeds, almond milk, and honey (if desired).
- Layer chia seed mixture and mixed berries in serving glasses.
- Refrigerate for at least 4 hours or overnight.

Nutrition Per Serving: Calories: 150 | Protein: 3g | Carbohydrates: 20g | Fiber: 7g | Fat: 7g

Chocolate Avocado Mousse

Preparation Time: 10 minutes | Cooking Time: 0 minutes | Total Time: 10 minutes | Number of Servings: 4

Ingredients:

- 2 ripe avocados

- 1/4 cup unsweetened cocoa powder
- 1/4 cup honey or maple syrup
- 1 teaspoon vanilla extract

Directions:

- Blend avocados, cocoa powder, honey, and vanilla extract until smooth.
- Serve as a creamy and guilt-free chocolate mousse.

Nutrition Per Serving: Calories: 200 | Protein: 2g | Carbohydrates: 20g | Fiber: 6g | Fat: 15g

Baked Apples with Cinnamon

Preparation Time: 10 minutes| Cooking Time: 40 minutes| Total Time: 50 minutes| Number of Servings: 4

Ingredients:

- 4 apples, cored and halved
- 1/4 cup chopped walnuts
- 1 teaspoon ground cinnamon
- 1/4 cup honey or maple syrup

Directions:

- Preheat the oven to 350°F (175°C).
- In a bowl, mix chopped walnuts, cinnamon, and honey.
- Fill the apple halves with the walnut mixture.
- Bake until the apples are tender and fragrant.

Nutrition Per Serving: Calories: 180 | Protein: 2g | Carbohydrates: 40g | Fiber: 6g | Fat: 4g

Coconut and Date Energy Balls

Preparation Time: 15 minutes| Cooking Time: 0 minutes| Total Time: 15 minutes| Number of Servings: 12

Ingredients*:*

- 1 cup pitted dates
- 1 cup shredded coconut
- 1/4 cup unsweetened cocoa powder
- 1/4 cup almond butter

Directions*:*

- In a food processor, blend dates, shredded coconut, cocoa powder, and almond butter until a sticky dough forms.
- Roll the mixture into small balls.
- Refrigerate to firm up.

Nutrition Per Serving (1 ball): Calories: 100 | Protein: 2g | Carbohydrates: 14g | Fiber: 3g | Fat: 5g

Mixed Berry Sorbet

Preparation Time: 10 minutes| Cooking Time: 0 minutes| Total Time: 2 hours (for freezing)| Number of Servings: 4

Ingredients*:*

- 2 cups mixed berries (blueberries, strawberries, raspberries)
- 1/4 cup honey or maple syrup
- Juice of 1 lemon

Directions:

- Blend mixed berries, honey or maple syrup, and lemon juice until smooth.
- Pour the mixture into a freezer-safe container.
- Freeze for at least 2 hours, stirring occasionally.

Nutrition Per Serving: Calories: 80 | Protein: 1g | Carbohydrates: 20g | Fiber: 3g | Fat: 0g

Watermelon and Mint Popsicles

Preparation Time: 10 minutes| Cooking Time: 0 minutes| Total Time: 4 hours (for freezing)| Number of Servings: 6

Ingredients:

- 4 cups diced watermelon
- Fresh mint leaves

Directions:

- Blend the diced watermelon until smooth.
- Pour the mixture into popsicle molds, adding fresh mint leaves.
- Freeze for at least 4 hours.

Nutrition Per Serving: Calories: 40 | Protein: 1g | Carbohydrates: 10g | Fiber: 1g | Fat: 0g

Banana and Peanut Butter Ice Cream

Preparation Time: 10 minutes| Cooking Time: 0 minutes| Total Time: 4 hours (for freezing)| Number of Servings: 4

Ingredients*:*

- 4 ripe bananas, sliced and frozen
- 1/4 cup natural peanut butter
- 1 teaspoon pure vanilla extract

Directions*:*

- Blend frozen banana slices, peanut butter, and vanilla extract until creamy.
- Freeze for at least 4 hours, then serve as healthy ice cream.

Nutrition Per Serving: Calories: 150 | Protein: 4g | Carbohydrates: 25g | Fiber: 3g | Fat: 5g

Dark Chocolate-Dipped Strawberries

Preparation Time: 10 minutes| Cooking Time: 5 minutes| Total Time: 15 minutes| Number of Servings: 4

Ingredients*:*

- 1 cup dark chocolate chips (70% cocoa or higher)
- 1 pint of fresh strawberries

Directions*:*

- Melt the dark chocolate chips in a microwave or over a double boiler.
- Dip each strawberry into the melted chocolate and place it on parchment paper.
- Allow the chocolate to harden before serving.

Nutrition Per Serving (4 strawberries): Calories: 100 | Protein: 2g | Carbohydrates: 15g | Fiber: 3g | Fat: 5g

Lemon Sorbet with Basil

Preparation Time: 15 minutes| Cooking Time: 0 minutes| Total Time: 2 hours (for freezing)| Number of Servings: 4

Ingredients*:*

- 1 cup fresh lemon juice
- Zest of 1 lemon
- 1/2 cup honey or maple syrup
- Fresh basil leaves

Directions*:*

- Mix lemon juice, lemon zest, and honey or maple syrup until well combined.
- Freeze for at least 2 hours, stirring occasionally, and garnish with fresh basil leaves before serving.

Nutrition Per Serving: Calories: 80 | Protein: 0g | Carbohydrates: 20g | Fiber: 0g | Fat: 0g

Pumpkin Spice Bites

Preparation Time: 20 minutes | Cooking Time: 0 minutes | Total Time: 20 minutes | Number of Servings: 12

Ingredients:

- 1 cup rolled oats
- 1/2 cup pumpkin puree
- 1/4 cup almond butter
- 1/4 cup honey or maple syrup
- 1 teaspoon pumpkin pie spice

Directions:

- In a bowl, mix rolled oats, pumpkin puree, almond butter, honey or maple syrup, and pumpkin pie spice.
- Roll the mixture into bite-sized balls.
- Refrigerate for a few minutes to firm up.

Nutrition Per Serving (1 bite): Calories: 70 | Protein: 2g | Carbohydrates: 10g | Fiber: 1g | Fat: 3g

APPENDICES

Glossary of Terms

1. **Acupuncture:** A traditional Chinese medicine technique involving the insertion of very thin needles through the skin at strategic points on the body, primarily used for pain relief and overall wellness.

2. **Antioxidants:** Substances that can prevent or slow damage to cells caused by free radicals, unstable molecules that the body produces as a response to environmental and other pressures.

3. **Ayurveda:** An ancient Indian system of medicine that uses a range of treatments, including herbal medicine, dietary changes, and yoga, to maintain or restore health.

4. **Bioflavonoids:** A group of plant compounds, found in fruits and vegetables, known for their antioxidant and anti-inflammatory health benefits.

5. **Chiropractic:** A form of alternative medicine mainly concerning the diagnosis and treatment of mechanical disorders of the musculoskeletal system, especially the spine.

6. **Detoxification:** The process of removing toxic substances or qualities. In terms of natural health, it often refers to diets, herbs, and other methods used to rid the body of toxins.

7. **Homeopathy:** A medical system based on the belief that the body can cure itself. It uses tiny amounts of natural substances, like plants and minerals, to treat the body.

8. **Naturopathy:** A form of alternative medicine employing a wide array of natural treatments, including herbalism, and acupuncture, along with diet and lifestyle counseling.

9. **Phytochemicals:** Chemical compounds produced by plants, generally to help them thrive or thwart competitors, predators, or pathogens. They can have health benefits when consumed.

10. **Probiotics:** Live bacteria and yeasts that are good for your health, especially your digestive system, often referred to as "good" or "helpful" bacteria.

11. **Qi (or Chi):** In traditional Chinese medicine, the life force or vital energy that flows

through the body, is usually manipulated through acupuncture and other practices.

12. **Reiki:** A form of alternative therapy commonly referred to as energy healing. It involves the transfer of energy by laying on hands.

13. **Superfoods**: Nutrient-rich foods are considered to be especially beneficial for health and well-being. They are often high in antioxidants, vitamins, and minerals.

14. **Tincture**: A concentrated herbal extract made by soaking herbs in alcohol or vinegar. Tinctures are used to deliver herbal benefits in a more potent form.

15. **Yoga**: An ancient practice that involves physical postures, breath control, and meditation, used to improve physical and mental well-being.

16. **Holistic**: A form of healing that considers the whole person — body, mind, spirit, and emotions — in the quest for optimal health and wellness.

17. **Inflammation**: The body's response to injury or infection, often causing redness, swelling,

warmth, and pain. Chronic inflammation is linked to various diseases.

18. **Macrobiotic Diet**: A diet based on the idea of balancing yin and yang elements in food, typically involving whole grains, vegetables, and beans.

19. **Oxidative Stress**: An imbalance between free radicals and antioxidants in the body, which can lead to cell and tissue damage.

20. **Reflexology**: A therapy based on the principle that there are reflex points on the feet, hands, and head linked to every part of the body.

21. **Veganism**: A diet and lifestyle that excludes all animal products and by-products, often motivated by health, ethical, or environmental concerns.

22. **Whole Foods**: Foods that are minimally processed and as close to their natural form as possible. They are typically free from artificial additives.

23. **Zinc**: A mineral important for immune function, wound healing, and DNA synthesis.

It's found in a variety of foods, including legumes, nuts, and seeds.

24. **Functional Medicine**: An approach that focuses on identifying and addressing the root cause of diseases, considering how various body systems interact.

25. **Meditation**: A practice where an individual uses a technique – such as mindfulness, or focusing the mind on a particular object, thought, or activity – to train attention and awareness, and achieve a mentally clear and emotionally calm state.

26. **Aromatherapy**: The use of essential oils extracted from plants for therapeutic purposes. It's believed to enhance physical and emotional health.

27. **Chelation Therapy**: A treatment used to remove heavy metals from the body, which involves the administration of chelating agents to bind and remove the metals.

28. **Essential Oils**: Highly concentrated plant extracts used in aromatherapy and other natural health practices. They are known for their aromatic and therapeutic properties.

29. **Fermentation**: A metabolic process that converts sugar to acids, gases, or alcohol. Fermented foods like yogurt and sauerkraut are rich in probiotics.

30. **Glycemic Index**: A number associated with the carbohydrates in a particular type of food that indicates the food's effect on a person's blood glucose (blood sugar) level.

31. **Hydrotherapy**: The use of water in various forms and at various temperatures for health purposes. This includes baths, saunas, steam rooms, and foot baths.

32. **Integrative Medicine**: A holistic approach to care that combines conventional medical treatments with complementary and alternative therapies.

33. **Kinesiology**: The scientific study of human or non-human body movement. In Complementary medicine, it refers to muscle-testing techniques used to diagnose imbalances in the body.

34. **Lymphatic Drainage**: A therapeutic massage treatment that uses gentle massage techniques to stimulate the circulation of lymph fluid around the body.

35. **Microbiome**: The collection of all the microorganisms living in association with the human body, including bacteria, viruses, and fungi, which play a crucial role in health and disease.

36. **Nutraceutical**: A product derived from food sources with extra health benefits in addition to the basic nutritional value found in foods.

37. **Osteopathy**: A type of alternative medicine that emphasizes physical manipulation of the body's muscle tissue and bones.

38. **Phytonutrients**: Natural compounds found in plants. They're known for their disease-preventing properties and are often found in fruits, vegetables, grains, and legumes.

39. **Qi Gong**: A holistic system of coordinated body posture and movement, breathing, and meditation used for health, spirituality, and martial arts training.

40. **Raw Food Diet**: A diet consisting mainly or entirely of raw and unprocessed foods. Advocates believe that cooking food decreases its nutritional value and enzyme content.

41. **Superbugs**: Strains of bacteria that have become resistant to antibiotic drugs. The rise of superbugs is a significant concern in modern medicine.

42. **Traditional Chinese Medicine (TCM)**: A traditional medical system originating in China that includes various forms of herbal medicine, acupuncture, massage (tui na), exercise (qi gong), and dietary therapy.

43. **Vitalism**: The belief in the existence of a vital force or life energy that animates living organisms, often a core concept in many traditional healing systems.

44. **Whole Grain**: Grains that contain all essential parts and naturally occurring nutrients of the entire grain seed. Examples include whole wheat, brown rice, and oats.

45. **Biodynamic Agriculture**: An advanced form of organic farming that emphasizes the holistic development and interrelationships of the soil, plants, and animals as a self-sustaining system. It often involves following an agricultural calendar and using specific compost preparations.

46. **Cryotherapy**: The use of extreme cold in medical therapy to treat a variety of tissue lesions, reduce inflammation, and alleviate pain. This can include methods like ice packs, coolant sprays, and whole-body cryotherapy chambers.

47. **Energetic Medicine**: A branch of complementary and alternative medicine that operates on the belief that a vital energy or life force flows through and around the body, influencing health. Treatments aim to balance this energy for physical and emotional well-being.

48. **Functional Foods**: Foods that have a potentially positive effect on health beyond basic nutrition. These foods may provide additional benefits that can reduce the risk of disease or promote optimal health. Examples include oats (for their fiber content), fatty fish (for omega-3 fatty acids), and probiotic-rich yogurt.

49. **Mindfulness**: A mental state achieved by focusing one's awareness on the present moment, while calmly acknowledging and accepting one's feelings, thoughts, and bodily sensations. It's often used as a

therapeutic technique to reduce stress and improve mental health.

50. **Nutritional Genomics**: The scientific study of the interaction between nutrition and genes, especially about the prevention or treatment of disease. It includes understanding how individual genetic makeup can affect the body's response to different nutrients.

This glossary is not exhaustive but provides a foundational understanding of many terms and concepts you will encounter in the field of natural health. It's designed to be a quick reference to help demystify complex terms and enhance your comprehension of the book's content.

DIRECTORY OF HERBS AND SUPPLEMENTS

Welcome to the Directory of Herbs and Supplements, a comprehensive guide to some of nature's most powerful healing agents. In this section, we'll delve into various herbs and supplements, exploring their traditional uses, potential health benefits, and how they might be incorporated into your wellness routine. Remember, while natural remedies can be potent allies in maintaining health and treating illness, it's always wise to consult with a healthcare professional before starting any new supplement or herbal regimen, especially if you have existing health conditions or are on medication.

1. Turmeric (Curcumin):

- **Traditional Uses:** Often used in Ayurvedic medicine for its anti-inflammatory properties.

- **Health Benefits:** May reduce inflammation, improve brain function, and lower the risk of heart disease.

- **Usage Tips:** These can be added to foods, taken as a supplement, or used in tea. Combining with black pepper enhances absorption.

2. Ginger:

- **Traditional Uses:** Widely used for digestive ailments.

- **Health Benefits:** Helps with nausea, and digestion, and may have anti-inflammatory and antioxidant effects.

- **Usage Tips:** Can be consumed fresh, as a dried spice, in tea, or as a supplement.

3. Garlic:

- **Traditional Uses:** Historically used for its medicinal properties.

- **Health Benefits:** May improve heart health, provide immune support, and have anti-cancer properties.

- **Usage Tips:** Best consumed fresh to maximize its benefits.

4. Echinacea:

- **Traditional Uses:** Commonly used to prevent colds and other respiratory infections.

- **Health Benefits:** Thought to boost the immune system.

- **Usage Tips:** Available as teas, capsules, and tinctures. Best taken at the onset of cold symptoms.

5. Ginseng:

- **Traditional Uses:** A staple in traditional Chinese medicine for energy and wellness.

- **Health Benefits:** May improve energy levels, reduce stress, and enhance brain function.

- **Usage Tips:** Available in capsules, teas, and extracts. Should be taken in cycles for the best results.

6. Omega-3 Fatty Acids (Fish Oil):

- **Traditional Uses:** Not traditionally used but recognized for heart health in modern times.

- **Health Benefits:** Supports heart health, and mental health, and reduces inflammation.

- **Usage Tips:** Available in capsules or liquid. It's important to ensure high purity to avoid heavy metal contamination.

7. Probiotics:

- **Traditional Uses:** Probiotics are more of a modern concept, but fermented foods have long histories.

- **Health Benefits:** Supports gut health, which can impact overall health, including the immune system.

- **Usage Tips:** Available as supplements or can be consumed in fermented foods like yogurt, kefir, and sauerkraut.

8. St. John's Wort:

- **Traditional Uses:** Used for mental health and mood disorders.

- **Health Benefits:** May help with mild to moderate depression.

- **Usage Tips:** Available in capsules, teas, and tinctures. Interacts with many medications, so consult a healthcare provider before use.

9. Green Tea Extract:

- **Traditional Uses:** Green tea has been consumed for centuries for its health benefits.

- **Health Benefits:** High in antioxidants, may aid in weight loss and improve brain function.

- **Usage Tips:** Can be consumed as tea or as a supplement in extract form.

10. Milk Thistle:

- **Traditional Uses:** Traditionally used to support liver health.

- **Health Benefits:** Believed to protect the liver from toxins and promote liver regeneration.

- **Usage Tips:** Available in capsules, teas, or as a liquid extract.

11. Ashwagandha:

- **Traditional Uses:** An important herb in Ayurvedic medicine for stress reduction and vitality.

- **Health Benefits:** May help reduce stress and anxiety, improve brain function, and boost energy levels.

- **Usage Tips:** Available in capsules, powders, and as a liquid extract.

12. Hawthorn Berry:

- **Traditional Uses:** Long used for heart health.

- **Health Benefits:** May improve cardiovascular function and reduce symptoms of heart failure.

- **Usage Tips:** Available as capsules, teas, or liquid extracts.

13. Ginkgo Biloba:

- **Traditional Uses:** An ancient tree used for cognitive health.

- **Health Benefits:** May improve memory and brain function, and enhance blood circulation.

- **Usage Tips:** Commonly taken in capsule or tablet form.

14. Valerian Root:

- **Traditional Uses:** Used for its sedative properties.

- **Health Benefits:** Often used as a natural treatment for sleep disorders and anxiety.

- **Usage Tips:** Available as capsules, teas, or tinctures.

15. Chamomile:

- **Traditional Uses:** Commonly used for relaxation and sleep.

- **Health Benefits:** May help with sleep issues, reduce menstrual pain, and act as an anti-inflammatory.

- **Usage Tips:** Commonly consumed as tea or taken as a supplement.

16. Saw Palmetto:

- **Traditional Uses:** Traditionally used for urinary symptoms.

- **Health Benefits:** May support prostate health and urinary function.

- **Usage Tips:** Usually taken in capsule form.

17. Aloe Vera:

- **Traditional Uses:** Widely used for skin conditions and digestive health.

- **Health Benefits:** May help with skin healing and gastrointestinal issues.

- **Usage Tips:** This can be used topically or consumed as a juice.

18. Flaxseed:

- **Traditional Uses:** Not traditionally used as a remedy, but recognized for its health benefits in modern times.

- **Health Benefits:** High in omega-3 fatty acids, and fiber, and may reduce cancer risk.

- **Usage Tips:** Can be added to foods in whole or ground form, or taken as an oil supplement.

19. Maca Root:

- **Traditional Uses:** Used in traditional Peruvian medicine for endurance and vitality.

- **Health Benefits:** May boost energy, improve mood, and enhance sexual health.

- **Usage Tips:** Available in powder, capsule, and liquid forms.

20. Spirulina:

- **Traditional Uses:** A type of blue-green algae used for nutritional purposes.

- **Health Benefits:** High in nutrients, may boost the immune system and improve cholesterol levels.

- **Usage Tips:** Available in tablet, powder, and capsule forms.

21. Black Cohosh:

- **Traditional Uses:** Commonly used for women's health issues.

- **Health Benefits:** May help with menopause symptoms like hot flashes and mood swings.

- **Usage Tips:** Generally taken in capsule or tincture form.

22. Rhodiola Rosea:

- **Traditional Uses:** Used for stress and stamina in traditional medicine.

- **Health Benefits:** May improve stress response, fatigue, and mental performance.

- **Usage Tips:** Available in capsule or tablet form.

23. Bilberry:

- **Traditional Uses:** Traditionally used for eye health and circulation.

- **Health Benefits:** May improve vision and support blood vessel health.

- **Usage Tips:** Available as capsules, teas, or extracts.

24. Milk Thistle:

- **Traditional Uses:** Used for liver health.

- **Health Benefits:** May protect the liver, promote liver regeneration, and help detoxify the body.

- **Usage Tips:** Available in capsules, teas, or liquid extracts.

25. Peppermint:

- **Traditional Uses:** Commonly used for digestive issues.

- **Health Benefits:** May help with IBS symptoms, nausea, and headaches.

- **Usage Tips:** Can be consumed as tea, capsules, or essential oil.

26. Licorice Root:

- **Traditional Uses:** Used for digestive health and respiratory issues.

- **Health Benefits:** May soothe gastrointestinal problems and respiratory infections.

- **Usage Tips:** Available as tea, capsules, or chewable tablets.

27. Dandelion:

- **Traditional Uses:** Historically used for liver and kidney health.

- **Health Benefits:** May support detoxification, improve liver function, and act as a diuretic.

- **Usage Tips:** Can be consumed as tea, in salads, or as a supplement.

28. Feverfew:

- **Traditional Uses:** Used for headache relief, particularly migraines.

- **Health Benefits:** May reduce migraine frequency and severity.

- **Usage Tips:** Available in capsules, tablets, and as a dried herb for tea.

29. Holy Basil (Tulsi):

- **Traditional Uses:** Important in Ayurvedic medicine for stress relief and overall wellness.

- **Health Benefits:** May reduce stress, improve mood, and support immune health.

- **Usage Tips:** Can be consumed as a tea or in capsule form.

30. Lemon Balm:

- **Traditional Uses:** Used for calming effects and to improve mood.

- **Health Benefits:** May help with anxiety, insomnia, and digestive issues.

- **Usage Tips:** Commonly taken as tea, capsules, or tinctures.

This comprehensive list provides a wide spectrum of herbs and supplements, each with its unique properties and potential health benefits. As you explore these natural remedies, always prioritize safety and informed decision-making. Remember, the key to effectively using these supplements is to understand your own health needs and to seek guidance from healthcare professionals when necessary.

RESOURCE GUIDE FOR FURTHER READING

Books and Literature

Barbara Oneill's Self-Heal By Design-

This book is a valuable resource for anyone looking to embrace a more natural, holistic approach to health and wellness.

Other Readings

1. **"The Encyclopedia of Natural Medicine" by Michael T. Murray and Joseph Pizzorno**

   - This comprehensive guide offers a deep dive into natural medicine. It covers a wide range of topics and provides detailed information on how to use natural remedies safely and effectively.

2. **"The Herbal Medicine-Maker's Handbook: A Home Manual" by James Green**

   - If you're interested in making your herbal remedies, this book is a treasure trove. It's practical, easy to understand, and filled with useful tips.

3. **"Healing With Whole Foods: Asian Traditions and Modern Nutrition" by Paul Pitchford**

   - This book is a blend of modern research and ancient wisdom. It gives insights into how foods affect our health and how we can use them to prevent and treat various diseases.

4. **"The Complete Book of Ayurvedic Home Remedies" by Vasant Lad**

   - Ayurveda, the ancient Indian system of medicine, offers a holistic approach to health. This book is a great starting point for anyone interested in exploring Ayurvedic remedies.

Online Resources

1. **National Center for Complementary and Integrative Health (NCCIH)**

   - [Website: nccih.nih.gov]

   - This government website offers reliable, research-based information on various complementary health approaches.

2. **The Herbal Academy**

   - [Website: theherbalacademy.com]

   - An excellent resource for those interested in learning about herbalism. They offer online courses ranging from beginner to advanced levels.

3. **NutritionFacts.org**

   - [Website: nutritionfacts.org]

   - Founded by Dr. Michael Greger, this non-profit site provides the latest in evidence-based nutrition research.

Podcasts and Video Channels

1. **"The Doctor's Farmacy" with Dr. Mark Hyman**

   - A podcast where Dr. Hyman discusses different aspects of functional medicine and holistic health.

2. **"Wellness Mama"**

   - A YouTube channel and website with a focus on natural health, recipes, and home remedies for families.

CONCLUSION

As we draw this journey to a close, let's reflect on the incredible landscape of natural remedies and self-healing we've traversed. This book was a voyage into the heart of healing, where nature's bounty meets human ingenuity, offering hope and health to those grappling with diseases like cancer, heart conditions, and diabetes.

We began by laying the foundations of health, emphasizing that true wellness is not just the absence of disease, but a harmonious balance of mind, body, and spirit. Nutrition, hydration, sleep, and exercise were spotlighted as the cornerstones of this balance, essential for fostering an environment where healing can flourish.

The power of foods and herbs in combating and managing diseases can't be overstated. We delved into how certain foods and herbs act as natural warriors against illness. Superfoods, anti-inflammatory ingredients, and heart-healthy diets are not just buzzwords; they are tools in our arsenal for fighting disease and boosting our overall health.

But it's not just about what we eat. We explored the holistic side of healing – the importance of detoxification, stress management, and alternative therapies. These elements play a pivotal role in aligning our physical health with our mental and emotional well-being. Techniques like meditation, acupuncture, and naturopathy aren't just alternative options; they are complementary to our health journey, offering benefits that often go beyond the physical.

As we navigated through the chapters dedicated to cancer, heart disease, and diabetes, it became evident that while each condition is unique, they all share a common thread - the potential for improvement through natural means. Integrating nutritional support, lifestyle changes, and natural supplements into treatment plans can offer a beacon of hope and a path toward better health.

The prevention strategies outlined in this book are not just about dodging diseases. They're about empowering ourselves to take charge of our health, to live not in fear of illness but in the celebration of wellness. Prevention is about making small, sustainable changes today that will pay dividends in our future health.

In crafting your natural remedy plan, remember that this journey is deeply personal. What works for one may not work for another. It's about listening to your body, understanding its needs, and responding with love and care.

As you close this book, remember that the health journey is ongoing. There's always more to learn, more to explore, and more ways to nurture your body and soul. The pursuit of health is not a destination but a path we walk every day. May this book be a companion on your journey, a guide amidst the complexities of the disease, and a beacon of hope in your quest for health.

So, take these lessons, embrace the natural remedies, and step forward into a life of enriched health and wellness. Here's to your health, naturally.

Printed in Great Britain
by Amazon